first place 4health

Bible Study Series

balanced living

Published by First Place 4 Health
Houston, Texas, U.S.A.
www.firstplace4health.com
Printed in the U.S.A.

All Scripture quotations are taken from the *Holy Bible, New International Version*®, NIV®
Copyright © 1973, 1978, 1984, 2011 by Biblica, Inc. Used by permission of Zondervan.
All rights reserved worldwide. www.zondervan.com The "NIV" and "New International
Version" are trademarks registered in the United States Patent and Trademark Office by Biblica, Inc.

©2014, 2010 First Place 4 Health. All rights reserved.
ISBN 978-1-942425-00-7

Caution: The information contained in this book is intended to be solely for
informational and educational purposes. It is assumed that the First Place 4 Health
participant will consult a medical or health professional before beginning this or
any other weight-loss or physical fitness program.

It is illegal to copy any part of this document without
permission from First Place 4 Health.

contents

Foreword by Carole Lewis 4

Introduction 5

BIBLE STUDIES

Week One: Welcome to *Balanced Living* 7

Week Two: Bumpy Road 8

Week Three: Balance Beam 25

Week Four: Budgeting for Balance 41

Week Five: CEO Secrets 57

Week Six: Possibilities and Responsibilities 73

Week Seven: Lawful or Helpful 89

Week Eight: Designed by the Master 105

Week Nine: Living the Good Life 121

Week Ten: Your Weakness, God's Power 137

Week Eleven: Sin Cancelled by Love 151

Week Twelve: Time to Celebrate! 163

ADDITIONAL MATERIALS

Leader Discussion Guide 164

First Place 4 Health Menu Plans 176

First Place 4 Health Member Survey 205

Personal Weight and Measurement Record 207

Weekly Prayer Partner Forms 209

Live It Trackers 231

Let's Count Our Miles! 255

Scripture Memory Verses 257

foreword

Welcome to one of the best decisions you will ever make -- taking steps toward giving Christ first place in every area of your life. More than twenty years ago, I was introduced to First Place 4 Health by my mother-in-law out of concern for the welfare of her grandchildren. I was overweight and overwrought. God used that first Bible study to start me on my journey to health, wellness and a life of balance. It will only take you about fifteen to twenty minutes to work through each day's study, but in those few minutes, you will discover the deep truths of God's Word. An important element of each week's study will be the Scripture memory verse for the week. As you focus on the truths found in God's word, He will begin to change you from the inside out. We long for you to experience the freedom that comes from an intimate relationship with Jesus Christ. He will reveal His love for you through the reading of his word and through prayer. In Luke 4:18-19, Jesus taught through the book of Isaiah, "The spirit of the Lord is on me, because he has anointed me to proclaim good news to the poor. He has sent me to proclaim freedom for the prisoners and recovery of sight for the blind, to set the oppressed free, to proclaim the year of the Lord's favor." Good news! He sets us free! Whether it be the chains of compulsivity, addiction, gluttony, overeating, under eating or just plain unbelief. It is my prayer that you will discover freedom in Christ so you may experience life--and not a small life. He has promised an abundant life. God bless you as you begin this exciting journey toward a life of liberty.

Vicki Heath, First Place 4 Health National Director

LUKE 4:18-19

introduction

First Place 4 Health is a Christ-centered health program that emphasizes balance in the physical, mental, emotional and spiritual areas of life. The First Place 4 Health program is meant to be a daily process. As we learn to keep Christ first in our lives, we will find that He is the One who satisfies our hunger and our every need.

This Bible study is designed to be used in conjunction with the First Place 4 Health program but can be beneficial for anyone interested in obtaining a balanced lifestyle. The Bible study has been created in a five-day format, with the last two days reserved for reflection on the material studied. Keep in mind that the ultimate goal of studying the Bible is not only for knowledge but also for application and a changed life. Don't feel anxious if you can't seem to find the *correct* answer. Many times, the Word will speak differently to different people, depending on where they are in their walk with God and the season of life they are experiencing. Be prepared to discuss with your fellow First Place 4 Health members what you learned that week through your study.

There are some additional components included with this study that will be helpful as you pursue the goal of giving Christ first place in every area of your life:

- **Group Prayer Request Form:** This form is at the end of each week's study. You can use this to record any special requests that might be given in class.

- **Leader Discussion Guide:** This discussion guide is provided to help the First Place 4 Health leader guide a group through this Bible study. It includes ideas for facilitating a First Place 4 Health class discussion for each week of the Bible study.

- **Two Weeks of Menu Plans with Recipes:** There are 14 days of meals, and all are interchangeable. Each day totals 1,400 to 1,500 calories and includes snacks. Instructions are given for those who need more calories. An accompanying grocery list includes items needed for each week of meals.

First Place 4 Health Member Survey: Fill this out and bring it to your first meeting. This information will help your leader know your interests and talents.

- **Personal Weight and Measurement Record:** Use this form to keep a record of your weight loss. Record any loss or gain on the chart after the weigh-in at each week's meeting.

- **Weekly Prayer Partner Forms:** Fill out this form before class and place it into a basket during the class meeting. After class, you will draw out a prayer request form, and this will be your prayer partner for the week. Try to call or email the person sometime before the next class meeting to encourage that person.

- **Live It Trackers:** Your Live It Tracker is to be completed at home and turned in to your leader at your weekly First Place 4 Health meeting. The Tracker is designed to help you practice mindfulness and stay accountable with regard to your eating and exercise habits. Step-by-step instructions for how to use the Live It Tracker are provided in the *Member's Guide*.

- **Let's Count Our Miles!** A worthy goal we encourage is for you to complete 100 miles of exercise during your 12 weeks in First Place 4 Health. There are many activities listed on pages 255-256 that count toward your goal of 100 miles. When you complete a mile of activity, mark off the box listed on the Hundred Mile Club chart located on the inside of the back cover.

- **Scripture Memory Cards:** These cards have been designed so you can use them while exercising. It is suggested that you punch a hole in the upper left corner and place the cards on a ring. You may want to take the cards in the car or to work so you can practice each week's Scripture memory verse throughout the day.

- **Scripture Memory CD:** All 10 Scripture memory verses have been put to music at an exercise tempo in the CD at the back of this study. Use this CD when exercising or even when you are just driving in your car. The words of Scripture are often easier to memorize when accompanied by music.

Week 0

welcome to
Balanced Living

At your first group meeting for this session of First Place 4 Health, you will meet your fellow members, get an overview of your materials and find out what you can expect at weekly meetings. The majority of your class time will be spent learning about the four-sided person concept, the Live It Food Plan, and how change begins from the inside out. You will also have a chance to ask any questions about how to get the most out of First Place 4 Health. If possible, complete the Member Survey on page 205 before your first group meeting. The information that you give will help your leader tailor the next 12 weeks to the needs of the whole group.

Each weekly meeting begins with a weigh-in for members. This will allow you to track your progress over the 12-week session. Your Week One weigh-in/measurement will establish a baseline of comparison so that you can set healthy goals for this session. If you are apprehensive about weighing in every week, talk with your group leader about your concerns. He or she will have some options for you to consider that will make the weigh-in activity encouraging rather than stressful.

The day after your first meeting, begin Week Two of this Bible study. This session, you and your group will recognize areas of your life that are out of balance and learn God's way of regaining your equilibrium. As you open yourself to the truth of Scripture and share your hopes and struggles with the members of your group during the next 12 weeks, you'll find yourself becoming the healthy child of God you are designed to be!

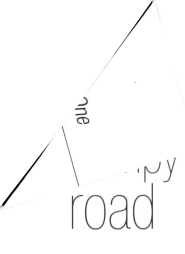

the happy road

SCRIPTURE MEMORY VERSE
This day I call heaven and earth as witnesses against you that I have set before you life and death, blessings and curses. Now choose life, so that you and your children may live.
DEUTERONOMY 30:19

Have you ever ridden in a vehicle whose wheels were out of balance? The car begins to vibrate when the car reaches 40 or so miles per hour, then increases at higher speeds and can be felt in the steering wheel, seats and floorboard. Instead of the tires spinning smoothly, they literally "bounce" down the road. The ride quality and comfort are poor, and the life of the tires, bearings, shocks and other components are much shorter than when the tires are kept in perfect balance.

Our lives sometimes get in the same shape as unbalanced wheels. At first we notice some vibration as we forge ahead without planning, and then the more we do and the faster we race through life, the louder and more intense the vibration becomes. Soon it's felt in our home, in our job, in our relationships and in our time with God. The quality of our life seems diminished, and we begin wearing out much faster than we would if we took steps to make small changes as we move forward on our journey through life.

Fixing unbalanced tires is easy: Just get the tires balanced! But what about our lives? How do we go about finding balance there? Is there a solution to out-of-balance eating? What do we do about one-sided thinking, uncontrolled emotions or loss of spiritual passion? This First Place

4 Health Bible study will help us understand and regain the balance that was intended for us by God in all four areas of our life: mental, physical, emotional and spiritual. Together with God, we will identify areas that lack balance and learn how to access and use His resources to live a healthier, longer and godlier lifestyle.

WHEEL ASSEMBLY • Day 1

Lord, as I begin this study, speak to my heart.
Be my guide and go with me as I travel. Amen.

A friend in the automotive repair business describes "wheel balance" as the proper distribution of weight around a revolving tire and wheel assembly. Proper wheel balance ensures that the wheels, while spinning, will not have heavy spots that will cause vibration as well as premature wear. Wheel balance is maintained by fitting tire weights to the rim of the wheel. Every time the tires are rotated, the wheels should also be checked for balance, as over time a weight may fall off while driving on rough roads or when making sharp turns.

In our life, as we head down rough roads, make sharp turns, or bad choices, we may lose sight of the weight (Jesus) in our life that keeps us balanced. Vibrations may show up in a relationship, job, overeating or other addictions. When it occurs in several areas at once, life becomes an uncomfortable ride. Draw a car wheel in the box below.

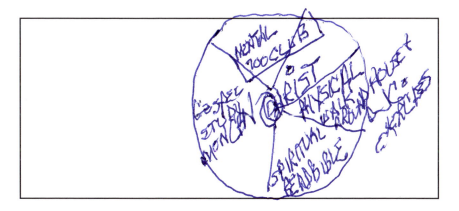

Consider this "wheel assembly" a visual of your life. Inside your wheel, write various activities and relationships that consume your time. What or who is at the center? Is there room for growing closer to God? In the space below, list activities you may choose to cut back on or eliminate to better balance your life.

_____

_____

_____

_____

In Ezekiel 36:26, God promised to give His people a new heart of flesh and remove the stony heart of sin. In Psalm 51:10, David considered his heart to be stony. Describe what David asked God for in that verse.

_____

_____

_____

Read Ezekiel 11:19-20. Verse 19 says: "I will give them an _____ heart and put a new _____ in them." An *undivided* heart is one free of addictions, materialism, immorality and self-indulgent behavior. In the space below or in your journal, list any activities on your wheel that divide your heart, squeezing God into the smallest space possible.

_____

_____

_____

_____

When God gives you a new heart of flesh and new desires, as He has promised, how do you think your life will change? What specific things will be different?

_____

_____

_____

According to this week's Scripture memory verse, God urges you to choose life. Think about some specific ways that you can choose life in each area of your life. Write your choices in the table below.

Physical	Mental
WALK MORE	*(handwritten)*
Spiritual	Emotional
	MEDITATE / READ BIBLE

Many vibrations that result from living an unbalanced life can be corrected by allowing God to replace your heart of stone with a heart of flesh. The journey is more enjoyable when God is driving, and we allow Him in the driver's seat when we have an undivided heart.

God, I have been traveling with unbalanced wheels. Give me a new heart of flesh and put Your Spirit within me. Amen.

BALANCING EQUIPMENT

Day 2

Heavenly Father, help me get my life in balance and teach me how to put You first so I can stay balanced. Be my foundation. Amen.

Balancing a wheel assembly must be done by a professional so that it is accurate and well-calibrated. How much more important is it that, in getting your life balanced, you use accurate equipment that measures accurately and comes to you from the best source? God provides equipment to help us balance all four areas of our life. God's truth in His Word will guide you toward a more balanced way of eating, handling emotional issues, growing strong in wisdom and in spiritual knowledge. He has given us Christian friends to support and encourage; His armor is available daily for protection; and gifts of the Spirit help us in our growth and service.

week two

What equipment has God provided to give you balance in each area of your life, and how are you using that equipment in your daily life?

Physical .

Emotional

Mental

Spiritual

There are many ways to include Bible reading into your daily life. You may start with the New Testament, reading one chapter or several verses each morning or evening. Find a plan that works for your schedule. How might this discipline help you achieve a more balanced life?

Hebrews 10:24 says, "Let us consider how we may spur one another on toward love and good deeds." How might you spur another class member on toward love and good deeds? Circle those activities you have already done and underline one you will try this week.

Make a phone call	Send an email	Pray together
Help with a problem	Mail a card	Practice memory verses

Whether you are a long-time First Place 4 Health member or are brand-new this session, establishing disciplines can enable you to reach your goals. Don't be afraid to ask for help in the areas where you are weak or to offer help when it's sought by others. Read the following Scripture verses and then write in your own words the kind of help each verse talks about.

Psalm 46:1
GOD IS ALWAYS WITH US TO PROVIDE STRENGTH AND SAFETY WE NEED ONLY ONLY TURN TO HIM AND HE

Isaiah 41:10
WILL HELP US SEEK & YE SHALL FIND ASK & IT SHALL BE GIVEN UNTO YOU

Psalm 121:8
HIS LOVE IS EVER PRESENT HE SHALL PRESERVE THY SOUL HE WILL KEEP YOU FROM ALL HARM HE WILL

Psalm 121 assures us that we can depend on God for help. Read that psalm, paying special attention to verses 7-8. How do you think the Lord can help you regain the balance you need for a healthier lifestyle? *HE WATCH OVER YOUR LIFE FROM YOUR GOING OUT AND YOUR COMING. IN PRESERVE THEE FROM ALL EVIL*

Vibrations that result from an out-of-balance life may appear in relationships, jobs, addictions and other areas of life. If you are experiencing vibrations, describe your situation and then share what you have learned today that gives you hope that those vibrations may be eliminated.

_____

_____

_____

_____

As you continue your weight-loss journey, the vibrations you experience may vary. There may be days you feel like parking the car and giving up. Don't! God is right there with you day and night, ready to get you back on the road toward reaching your goal.

Lord, thank You for supplying the proper equipment for a balanced life.
My help comes from You, and I want that strength within me. Amen.

Day 3 — HAVING A STANDARD

Thank You, Lord, for being with me through this week,
for giving me direction and for loving me when I seem to need it the most.
Help me grow strong and closer to You. Amen.

Some tires have marks on the tire sidewall to help auto repair professionals correctly balance the wheels. Aligning the marks assures that the tire has been properly mounted and will provide a smooth ride.

Similarly, we have a standard with which to align ourselves on our journey toward healthy eating and a more balanced lifestyle. Our standard is the Lord Jesus Christ. When our lives are lined up with Him, our eating is under control, our minds are free from self-deception, our relationships flourish and our walk with God is growing. God's Word is the place we find the standard for a healthy life. When we read, memorize, quote and apply Scripture to our life consistently, we become more in line with His Son.

bumpy road | 15

Write this week's memory verse, and then underline the action God commands you to do.

_____

_____

_____

God commands you to choose life for one simple reason: "So that _____ your _____ may _____." How is the First Place 4 Health program part of choosing life so that you and your children may live?

_____

_____

_____

Look up Hebrews 12:2-3. List several ways that you can "fix your eyes on Jesus" to help you on your weight-loss journey.

ME → SO MUCH OPPOSITION FROM SINNERS
SO THAT WOULD NOT GROW
WEARY + LOSE HEART

In verse 3 of Hebrews 12, we are told to consider Jesus, who endured so much, so that we won't grow weary and lose heart. Bringing balance into your life takes time; there may be days you feel overwhelmed. How does "considering Jesus" give you strength and encouragement?

THE REALITY OF WHAT JESUS
SUFFERED SO THAT WE
WOULD BE STRONG & NOT
LOSE HEART (HOPE

We have all felt weary at times, and may have resorted to unhealthy eating or withdrawing from others to make ourselves feel better. What is an area of your life in which you have felt the most weariness?

_____

_____

_____

Read Hebrews 12:2-3 again. Christ endured the cross and suffered terribly at the hands of sinful men. When we experience weariness, we can look at Jesus and consider how He never lost heart, never gave up and was never unfaithful to the Father. When we fix our eyes on Him, He becomes our example of persevering. Write a short prayer of thankfulness to Jesus for His willingness to endure so much for you.

Lord Jesus, having You in the center of my life is my standard. Help me focus on You by reading Your Word and applying it to my life. Amen.

Day 4 — FOLLOW MANUFACTURER INSTRUCTIONS

Lord God, help me to be obedient and walk in what I know is right. Keep me from turning away from You. Amen.

There are more wheel types than there are vehicles, so it is important to follow the manufacturer's instructions for proper mounting techniques. Obviously, the instructions for wheel mounting on a Honda sedan would not be the same as for a Chevy truck.

People are diverse as well. God made each of us unique—with different traits, gifts and features—and He works individually in our lives according to His plan for us. One type of instruction does not always work for everyone. Just because one way works in your neighbor's life doesn't mean that it will be effective in yours. When we follow God's instructions for our own life, our journey will be smoother and more enjoyable. It will also be an encouragement for others as they see God at work in us.

Read Psalm 139:13-16. According to verse 13, how were you created?

---

bumpy road | 17

Our Creator knit us together and stamped His image onto each of us. And not only that! When we put our trust in Jesus, His Holy Spirit resides in us to help us become all that God created us to be. Verse 14 gives us two reasons to praise God. What are they?

1. _____

2. _____

According to verse 15, what is not hidden from God?

_____

_____

_____

Our frame was not hidden from God before we were born; yet we sometimes try to hide it from Him now. How silly! He knew our failures and successes long before we did them. Is there anything you are still trying to hide from God? Why? How does acknowledging that God already knows make a difference?

_____

_____

_____

_____

Verse 16 begins with David recognizing something about God. What is it?

_____

_____

_____

David recognized that God saw his unformed body—everything God wanted him to have was already in him, even when David was in his mother's womb. Likewise, God saw your unformed body and had a vision of the good He could accomplish in and through you as well. How does knowing that change the way you view yourself and encourage you to take better care of His creation?

You are a marvelous creation made by an awesome God. By working together with Him to balance your thoughts and by following His instructions, you will learn to respect yourself, your body, the way God respects His creation . . . by loving it.

Father, discovering all that You see in me will take time. I know I am fearfully and wonderfully made, but sometimes it's difficult to see. Help me through this process. Thank You for loving me. Amen.

Day 5 — PREVENTING DAMAGE

Keep me safe, O God; protect me throughout the day. You are my refuge, the One I turn to for safekeeping. Amen.

With regular maintenance, tires last a lot longer and provide better quality performance. For this reason, most manufacturers suggest regularly cleaning deposits of foreign material from inside the wheel/rim and removing any stones from the tire tread. There are also special coatings that can be applied to a tire's finish to protect it from damage.

As you continue your weight-loss journey in First Place 4 Health, there is much you can do to prevent your life from sustaining damage. Cleaning out foreign materials is a good first step. Getting rid of fattening junk food and eliminating activities in your schedule that hinder you or drag you into temptation are preventative measures that will help you get where you want to go. List some of the things you are willing to clean out this week.

From your kitchen:

_____
_____
_____

From your schedule:

_____
_____
_____

From your mind:

_____
_____
_____

Each time you remove these "stones," the journey will get smoother. Yet you also need to protect the finish by putting on the full armor of God. Read Ephesians 6:11-17. Name each piece of the armor of God.

1. _____
2. _____
3. _____
4. _____
5. _____
6. _____

Read verse 14. Thinking in particular about your weight-loss efforts, describe how you can be protected from Satan's lies by wearing the belt of truth. How can memorizing Scripture protect you from enemy attacks?

_____
_____
_____
_____

This same verse mentions the breastplate of righteousness, which protects your heart. Satan often attacks our emotions, our feelings of self-worth or our ability to trust God and others. How can wearing the breastplate protect you from attacks on your heart?

_____

_____

_____

Verse 15 describes the shoes that represent a readiness to spread the gospel. Satan may attempt to convince you that no one will listen to your testimony because of your weight. If you have been tempted to believe his lies, how might the study from yesterday (Day 4) help?

_____

_____

_____

Verse 16 describes the shield of faith. How can you use your faith to ward off Satan's fiery darts of lies, insults and temptation?

_____

_____

_____

The helmet of salvation, described in verse 17, protects your mind from doubts about God and His love for you. List some ways that wearing your helmet can protect your mind.

_____

_____

_____

Also described in verse 17 is the only offensive weapon, the sword of the Spirit, the Word of God. By memorizing God's Word, you can defeat Sa-

tan's lies with God's truth. Have you memorized this week's Scripture
memory verse? Write it below.

When you put on all (not just some!) of God's armor, you are protected
against the spiritual forces of evil and are able to stand against the devil's
schemes. By spending time meditating and acting on God's Word, His
armor will help you overcome temptation and lead you into victory.

*Lord, I can't do this alone! Each morning, remind me to put on the full armor
so I will be protected as I move toward the goal You have for me. Amen.*

REFLECTION AND APPLICATION

Day
6

*Heavenly Father, You are the One I go to in prayer to share my thoughts,
needs and desires. Thank You for listening and answering. Amen.*

Driving a vehicle with out-of-balance wheels is not pleasant. At first, you
may barely notice the rough ride because it comes on slowly. But when the
steering wheel begins to vibrate, it is difficult to maintain control of the
car. The noise can give you a headache and cause embarrassment when
friends ride with you. Eventually, it is not safe to continue driving.

In the same way, we have to face the reality that out-of-balance eating is dangerous. Over the years, wrong choices didn't seem so bad; we'd
skip a meal and lose the extra pounds, or try a fad diet for a couple weeks,
only to go off of it and regain. The vibrations of an unbalanced life began getting louder and louder until we could no longer ignore the
threats to our health and other areas of life.

Have you noticed vibrations in any of the four areas of your life? Mental, physical, emotional or spiritual imbalance can cause an uncomfortable journey and will eventually become dangerous. Furthermore, finding
balance is not do-it-yourself. God will explore with you the reasons for

your imbalance, and provide resources to guide you toward making lifestyle changes.

Reflect on your "unbalanced wheels." In the space below or in your journal, share with God what you would like to see happen in your life. Make this a time of openness and honesty, remembering that God already knows where the imbalance is—He just wants you to become aware. Then listen as He shares with you what He has in store.

_____

_____

_____

_____

Lord, I want to be more balanced in all areas. Help me to make good choices, one day at a time, until my life reflects You, my Lord and Savior. Amen.

Day
7

REFLECTION AND APPLICATION

Those who seek You will find You. Show me Your desire for my life today and empower me to follow Your instructions and plan for my journey. Amen.

This week, you began the process of getting your wheels balanced by identifying the areas of vibration in your life. Looking at your heart as a wheel allowed you to see what/who is at the center. You discovered on Day 2 that God has provided everything you need to succeed. Think about and describe some of God's resources that you can put into use today that will help you move forward, remain strong and be encouraged.

_____

_____

_____

_____

On Day 4, you discovered in Psalm 139 how unique you are and how God deals with each of us individually. Seeing God's vision for your life is important for becoming emotionally healthy. List at least one good quality that God created in you for each area (mental, physical, emotional, spiritual), and read them throughout the coming week.

Physical

_____

_____

_____

Emotional

_____

_____

_____

Mental

_____

_____

_____

Spiritual

_____

_____

_____

On an index card, draw a wheel as you did on Day 1, but divide it the way you feel God would like you to balance each area of your life. Take time to pray, asking God to help you move from the first circle toward the second. It won't happen overnight; rather, it will be a slow, steady process that will unfold throughout your life. Post the card where you will see it daily to help you line up to the mark of Jesus Christ.

Heavenly Father, thank You for loving me even when I make choices that are not Your plan for my life. Forgive me when I allow my life to become unbalanced. I want to live my life with a healthy body, mind, soul and spirit. Amen.

Group Prayer Requests

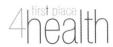

Today's Date: _____

Name	Request

Results

Week Three

balance
beam

SCRIPTURE MEMORY VERSE
*Jesus grew in wisdom and stature,
and in favor with God and men.*
LUKE 2:52

In 1996, the US women's gymnastic team was close to winning Olympic gold, but had one more event: the vault. Kerri Strug, who was 18 years old, was the last gymnast to compete. On her first attempt, she injured her ankle; the situation did not look good for the American team. But Kerri stuck her second vault's landing before the injury brought her down in pain, bringing home the gold for the American team.

Watching the Olympics is exciting; when all goes right, gymnasts mount the balance beam, perform with precision and dismount flawlessly in arm-raising victory. It may look effortless, but the success we witness as spectators depends on the gymnasts' ability to find balance. They train physically by putting in untold hours of training, learning to prioritize and make hard choices from a very early age. Saying no, even to good things, is part of the discipline they learn in order to succeed at their chosen sport. They maintain healthy bodies to endure the physical strain of competition, and often forego social time with friends and family in order to achieve their dream. Winning requires balance in all areas of life: mental, physical, spiritual and emotional.

This week, we will look at the different ways athletes must train in order to bring home the gold, and discover how we can apply similar disciplines to help us move toward a more balanced life.

26 | week three

Day 1 PREPARING MENTALLY

Lord, prepare my mind for the truth You are about to give me through Your Word and help me use it today. Amen.

Gymnasts prepare mentally long before they attempt a mount. They begin by adopting a "winner's mindset." Athletes must truly believe that they can win. Keeping a vision of the Olympic medals in their minds keeps them focused on the reward to come. Medals are the driving force for them when things go wrong, when their bodies get tired or when hope seems to fade. On days of discouragement, they recall that gleaming medal and all that it means as a way of staying in the game mentally.

Overweight people often have difficulty in developing a winner's mindset because they have failed so many times to lose weight and keep it off. Diets do not work over the long haul. A person loses weight, then gains it back, then loses and gains, until defeat sets in and that person becomes convinced that he or she will always be fat. First Place 4 Health is not a diet; it is a program for healthy, balanced living that will help you adopt a winner's mindset.

To prepare mentally to make lifestyle changes, you must believe it is doable. Forget what is past—because you can't change it—and focus on today. As you study God's Word, you will get a glimpse of how God sees you. He will begin transforming your mind and you will grow in wisdom, make wiser choices and move closer to your goal.

Read Romans 12:2. What are we told to do?

_____

_____

_____

What are we told *not* to do?

_____

_____

_____

How can you apply this Scripture to areas you struggle with the most?

The "pattern of this world" leads to obesity, along with many complications. What is one change you will make today in order not to conform to the world? (Remember that though Christians are living *in* this world, they are not *of* the world.)

The last part of Romans 12:2 explains what we will be able to do with a renewed mind. What is it?

The more we apply the truth of God's Word to our daily lives, the better we will understand God's will for us. When you allow God to transform you by renewing your mind, His will becomes your will. Memorizing Scripture verses will help you mount the balance beam, supporting you as you continue toward the prize. When things go wrong, when your body gets tired or when hope seems to fade, God will transform your mind through His Word so that you can say with conviction, "I can do all things through Christ who gives me strength" (Philippians 4:13).

Lord, my desire is to be like You. You are the prize I seek, and I know in my heart that You will give me the strength I need to obtain it. Amen.

28 | week three

Day 2

RESISTANCE EXERCISE

Father, today I set my mind on Your truth and ask that
You fill me with Your Holy Spirit that I might know Your will. Amen.

Many of us have practiced "resistance exercise" over the years; we have simply resisted exercise! We don't like to sweat or to endure the discomfort we encounter when muscles meet resistance. Yet true resistance training is absolutely necessary for a balanced life. Temptation requires resistance, whether it's getting out the door to walk or to spend time with the Lord instead of sleeping longer; saying no to a second helping or to a fast-food drive-thru; or struggling to memorize Scripture verses and to make time for daily Bible study.

Read 1 Corinthians 10:12-13. In verse 13, the apostle Paul reminds us that "no temptation has seized you except what is _____ to man." On days when you find that you are tempted to give in to temptation, you can be sure you are not alone. Paul goes on to give us good news in the remainder of verse 13:

> And God is faithful; he will not let you be tempted beyond what you can bear. But when you are tempted, he will also provide a way out so that you can stand up under it.

Describe in the space below how these phrases offer you encouragement.

_____

_____

_____

_____

Our lives are filled with inactivity, due in part to many laborsaving devices, resulting in our muscles rarely being pushed very hard. Raking leaves, mowing the lawn and washing the car by hand are tasks we do less often than generations before; elevators and escalators carry us to

balance beam | 29

various floors in stores and airports, and washing clothes and dishes are chores for machines. Add to that the inactive appeal of computers, electronic games, television and iPods, and you can understand why our muscles are deteriorating and obesity is increasing. Research has shown that physical inactivity is the second leading preventable cause of death in the United States.[1] It is literally killing us.

List four laborsaving devices you use on a regular basis.

1. _____
2. _____
3. _____
4. _____

Circle two of these that you are willing to resist using this week, replacing them with the physical labor required to perform the job. Next, thinking now of entertainment, write down four "inactive activities" that you engage in daily (video games, surfing the Internet, watching television, and so forth).

1. _____
2. _____
3. _____
4. _____

Now circle one of these that you are willing to resist using this week, and what you will replace it with (physical game, sport or activity). As we learn to resist inactivity, which causes our muscles to atrophy, and replace it with activities that benefit our bodies, we will become stronger. With exercise, something is better than nothing and more is better than less.

Lord Jesus, help me change my view of exercise. Help me go from resisting exercise to exercising resistance when temptations come into my life. Amen.

week three

Day 3

SPIRITUALLY SOUND

Jesus, my Savior, I love You and desire to follow after You.
Just for today, show me the path You want me to walk. Amen.

When a gymnast mounts a balance beam, her surefootedness is largely dependant on having a sound foundation. If that beam is unstable, too soft or hard, it will cause her to lose focus and possibly the competition. A solid foundation can mean the difference between a gold, silver or bronze medal—or no medal at all.

A gymnast competes to win; each one wants that gold medal, the ultimate prize. A Christian's ultimate prize is Jesus Christ, and following Him is also dependant on having a sure foundation.

Read 2 Timothy 2:19 and fill in the blanks.

Nevertheless, God's solid _____ stands _____, sealed with this inscription: "The _____ knows those who are _____," and, "Everyone who confesses the name of the _____ must _____ _____ from wickedness."

Describe the foundation we have when we confess Christ, according to the verse above. What does this foundation mean to you?

_____

_____

_____

_____

_____

Read 1 Corinthians 3:11. What is the foundation in this verse?

_____

_____

_____

_____

In Isaiah 28:16 the Lord says, "See, I lay a stone in Zion, a tested stone, a precious cornerstone for a sure foundation; the one who trusts will never be dismayed." That precious cornerstone is Jesus Christ. He is the one who makes the foundation sure and solid! Look again at the verse in Isaiah. Who will never be dismayed? What does he put his trust in?

_____

_____

_____

_____

Can you say in your heart that Jesus Christ is your foundation, that you have placed your trust in Him? In Romans 10:13, Paul says, "Everyone who calls on the name of the Lord will be saved." You can do that simply by asking Jesus to be your personal Savior. You might pray something like this:

> *Jesus, I believe that You are the Son of God and that You died for all my sins. I confess to You now that I have sinned and I ask Your forgiveness. I'm placing my trust in You to be saved. Please make my foundation sure. Forgive me and come into my heart. Be my Lord and Savior for all eternity. Amen.*

If you prayed the above prayer or one from your heart and received the gift of eternal life, please share that decision with your leader. You're off to a great start!

Perhaps you made that decision years ago, but have allowed your relationship with Jesus, your foundation, to fall into disrepair. Now is a good time to ask the Lord to help you begin working on any weak areas, to get rid of the cracks and crevices that allow temptations to enter into your life.

List three areas of weakness that you may have noticed in your life over the past several months, and then jot down which area(s) of your life it affects (physical, mental, emotional or spiritual). If you have difficulty with this, ask God to reveal to you what He wants you to see.

1. _____
2. _____
3. _____

Spend some time with God and share this with Him, asking for His help to strengthen those areas.

God, thank You for Your Son. I want to become spiritually sound,
and I know that unless I trust Jesus, my foundation won't be sure! Amen.

Day 4 TEAM PLAYER

Father, I am glad that I'm on Your team. Just knowing You are encouraging
me and watching over me gives me hope that I will have victory. Amen.

As part of a four-man relay swim competition in the 2008 Olympics, Michael Phelps broke his own record and was largely responsible for the U.S. taking home the gold medal. When Michael was interviewed on camera, he declared that the win came out of the willingness of the team to work together, with each man doing his part to the best of his ability.

We each must do our part to the best of our ability. We aren't competing against others in our group—only ourselves, trying to do better each week. We will have days when we do everything right, and then we will have days that we wish we could cut from the calendar. We practice what we know, use the tools we've been given and apply it to our lives.

The best part of being in a group is that you are not alone. You have a leader who wants to help you succeed, along with fellow members to offer encouragement and prayer—but God is your ultimate team member. He will support you during your journey. He wants to help you win the prize.

balance beam | 33

Read Romans 12:10. How might you work out this verse among others in your group?

_____

_____

_____

_____

When you do your part and work in tandem with God, you'll be able to declare that you won because of your willingness to work together with God, your leader and your fellow group members, while doing your part to the best of your ability.

Look up the following verses and draw a line from the reference to the correct content of the verse.

Acts 15:32	But encourage one another daily
Psalm 10:17	Let us not give up meeting together
Hebrews 3:13	Said much to encourage and strengthen
Romans 15:4-5	You encourage and listen to their cry
Hebrews 10:25	God gives endurance and encouragement

One of the benefits of being in your group is the encouragement you receive. When you do well, they celebrate with you; when you have difficult days, you receive their support in the form of prayer, cards and phone calls. The Scriptures you memorize are another form of support, along with communication with God during your daily quiet time. But being a team player means that *you* have a part to fulfill in providing that same encouragement for others. What does Paul remind us that we are to do in 2 Corinthians 1:3-5?

_____

_____

_____

_____

Have you done your part to the best of your ability? Think of someone in your group who needs encouragement. What are two things you can do this week to support him or her?

_____

_____

_____

_____

_____

Heavenly Father, I'm so glad You're on my team. Help me daily to become the best member I can be on Your team. Amen.

Day 5

IMPERFECT BALANCE

Lord, there are some days when I just can't seem to get it right and I fall short of what I know I should do. Thank You for Your love, mercy, grace and forgiveness during these times. Amen.

Think about how successful you would feel if you made all the right decisions—if you ate only what was healthy and became physically active; if you worshiped with your entire being, following the Lord in total obedience; and if you treated others the way you want to be treated. Knowing that we are all imperfect people and incapable of achieving perfection is no excuse for not moving toward what we could call "imperfect balance." Jesus was human, without sin—perfect. Striving to become more like Him every day is not an impossibility.

Write this week's memory verse below.

_____

_____

_____

_____

_____

Notice that this verse begins with the words "Jesus grew." Jesus grew when He went to the Temple, listened to the teachers and asked questions (see Luke 2:41-52). He used these learning opportunities to grow in all four areas of His life, balancing them so that He could fulfill God's plan for Him. His knowledge grew into wisdom. He became physically fit. His relationship with the Father was so intimate that He knew exactly what God expected of Him. He formed lasting and secure relationships with His closest friends, His disciples.

Getting your imperfect balancing act together happens over time, not overnight! Don't beat yourself up because you made a bad decision or overate at lunch. Don't berate yourself when you forget one morning to get up early enough to spend time with the Lord. If you have an argument with your spouse or friend, ask forgiveness from him or her and from God and move on. If any of it was your fault, then take responsibility and ask God to help you do better. Remember, "Jesus grew."

Read 2 Peter 3:18. What does the apostle Peter say you should do?

How can you begin doing this today in your life?

As you read and study the Word of God, you will grow into a more balanced life. Everything won't be perfect, but you will find that, over time, you will have more successes than losses on that balance beam of life.

Lord, help my imperfect balance reflect a daily improvement so that when I stand before You, I will know that I have done my best. Amen.

week three

Day 6

REFLECTION AND APPLICATION

Today, Lord, as I look back and see the choices I made during the week, help me to learn from my mistakes and teach me how to use discernment in the coming week. Amen.

Your balance-beam performance this week may or may not have gone as you hoped or planned. You may have mounted up easily, or you may have had to repeat that mount several times before finding a sure-footed stance without wavering.

The statement "showing up is half the battle" has some validity. You must show up, learn the basics, follow directions and take responsibility in order to mount the beam. Showing up is how you learn to find the perfect balance for your life. Your involvement in First Place 4 Health indicates your desire to show up, learn the basics, follow directions and take responsibility.

It doesn't matter where you are or how many times you have fallen. You are here now, and Jesus will meet you where you are. But He won't leave you there. He wants to teach you how to get your balance, one day at a time. He is your personal trainer, able to guide and support you as you become more like Him every day.

Ask yourself the following questions and write your answers here or in your journal.

What have I done mentally this week to stop conforming to the world's pattern regarding my health?

balance beam | 37

What physical activity have I started doing this week and how many times did I participate in it?

Have I made Jesus Christ my foundation?

How have I shown God and others that I am a team player?

In what ways have I chosen to grow more like Jesus this week?

Lord, show me Your ways, teach me Your paths; guide me in
Your truth and teach me, for You are God my Savior,
and my hope is in You all day long (see Psalm 25:4-5). Amen.

Day 7

REFLECTION AND APPLICATION

God, thank You for Your power and wisdom. I depend on You for everything. Having access to that power through prayer and the Holy Spirit keeps me moving forward. Amen.

You have probably noticed that after each day's *Balanced Living* study, there is a prayer. Hopefully, you have found these prayers helpful in connecting to God's awesome power within you. That power can be used to resist the devil and cause him to flee. It can strengthen you on weak days and build you up. God's power can bring you back into balance when things get off-kilter.

Many believers have practiced a prayer discipline in which they write God's Word in their own words as a prayer back to Him. Isaiah 55:11 says, "So is my word that goes out from my mouth: It will not return to me empty, but will accomplish what I desire and achieve the purpose for which I sent it." As you learn this wonderful prayer technique and establish the habit of praying God's word back to Him, your prayer life will come alive.

Look up the following Scriptures (or choose some of your own) and rewrite them in your own way in the form of a prayer. Then pray them back to God. (Look at the closing prayer below to get you started.) Choose verses that have special meaning to you or that offer promises of victory. Remember, God's Word will not return to Him without accomplishing its purpose.

1 Peter 5:8

_____

_____

_____

_____

_____

_____

balance beam | 39

Matthew 26:41

_____

_____

_____

_____

_____

_____

Isaiah 26:3

_____

_____

_____

_____

_____

_____

Lord, You say that life is more important than food and that my body is more important than clothes. Help me take my focus off of these things. I want my focus to be only on You (see Matthew 6:25). Amen.

Note

1. "CDC: Obesity Approaching Tobacco as Top Preventable Cause of Death," Doc torsLounge.com, April 5, 2004. http://www.doctorslounge.com/primary/arti cles/obesity_death/.

Group Prayer Requests

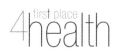

Today's Date: _____

Name	Request

Results

_____
_____
_____
_____
_____

Week Four

budgeting for balance

SCRIPTURE MEMORY VERSE

Be strong and very courageous. Be careful to obey all the law my servant Moses gave you; do not turn from it to the right or to the left, that you may be successful wherever you go.

JOSHUA 1:7

Trying to find balance doesn't just happen, any more than finding time to do all you need and want to do "just happens." You make time for what is important to you. In the same way, you must make time to learn how to balance the four areas of your life—mental, physical, spiritual and emotional. Budgeting for balance involves identifying, planning for and evaluating what is going on in your life. It is about discovery and prioritizing—finding what is wrong so that you can do what is right.

This week's study will provide hands-on, practical ways for you to begin balancing each area in your "life checkbook." It won't happen overnight, but gradually you will see improvement where before there was chaos. As this week's memory verse warns, you will need to be strong and very courageous; but learning the basics of budgeting is an adventure when you begin using it to keep a more balanced mental, physical, spiritual and emotional life.

Budgeting for balance in your life will enable you to see your life from God's perspective. He will help you adjust the scale so the weights you deal with are evenly distributed, more manageable and lightened—and possibly discarded altogether.

42 | week four

Day 1

IT TAKES COURAGE TO COUNT THE COST

Lord, help me to look at what is wrong in my life and give me the courage to work hard at making it right. Show me what I need to do and give me the strength to do it. Amen.

Budgeting is not always pleasant. It takes time and effort to work through areas that we have avoided addressing. Some people would rather just plunge in and hope for the best, thinking ignorance is bliss. But Joshua instructs us in our memory verse to be strong and very courageous. It takes courage to face your faults and learn to better manage your finances, time and other aspects of your life. Often, you must learn to say no (especially to things and people you love), when you want to say yes.

Read Luke 14:25-35. What two examples of counting the cost does Jesus describe?

1. _____

2. _____

Now think about your own life. Can you match the above examples with circumstances or relationships that you need to reevaluate or reprioritize?

1. _____

2. _____

Jesus asks two very similar questions in verses 28 and 31. Rewrite this question in your own words, so that it addresses a circumstance or relationship you noted above.

_____

_____

_____

_____

budgeting for balance | 43

If you want to have balance in your life, you must first identify how you are spending your time, energy and talents. You may be involved in many things that take away from your ability to be available for God and do nothing to help you achieve your goals—but how will you know unless you identify these activities? In your journal or below, identify activities and relationships you are involved in for each area of your life.

Mental

_____

_____

_____

_____

Physical

_____

_____

_____

_____

Spiritual

_____

_____

_____

_____

Fmotional

_____

_____

_____

_____

When you have completed the above exercise, go through your list and ask God how each activity and relationship fits into His plan for you.

Give this process time and plenty of prayer. When you sense God moving you, draw a line through any items on the list that need to be eliminated. Put a check mark next to activities or relationships that are church-related and circle those that involve job, family or friends. If there are hobby activities, underline them.

Perhaps you pay dues and attend a monthly business association meeting, but you find that you don't really benefit from it. Or, you might be president in a hobby club and realize that your involvement is consuming valuable amounts of your time. Give yourself permission to let some of these things fall away and to say no when asked to serve in an area that is unrelated to your life goals.

The goal here should be to please God rather than man (see Galatians 1:10). This process will help you begin focusing on your life goals and devoting more time to family, church and, most importantly, God.

Lord Jesus, my days seem to get swallowed up in busy-work, job, family, hobbies and relationships. My desire is to please You, not to win the approval of men. Help me discover what You have planned for my life. Amen.

Day 2
ADHERE TO YOUR PLAN

Show me Your plan for my journey, Lord, and empower me to stick to it instead of my own. Teach me what I need to learn and remind me to come to You for help. Amen.

A popular TV show in the 1980s was *The A-Team*, and one of the main characters, Colonel John "Hannibal" Smith, had a wonderful catch-phrase: "I love it when a plan comes together." It *does* feel good to work on a plan and have it all come together for success. Do plans always work out that way? Of course not—especially when you are working your own plan using worldly standards and direction, leaving God out of the picture. Your plan may look good on the page in your Day-Timer, but God sees it differently.

budgeting for balance | 45

Read Psalm 33:10-11. After reading this passage, why do you think God sometimes thwarts the plans people make?

_____

_____

_____

_____

Read Proverbs 20:18 and explain in your own words how we should make our plans.

_____

_____

_____

_____

When you seek God and get a plan in motion, you may still get side-tracked. Sometimes this occurs because other people or circumstances get in the way, but most often it is because you fail to stick to the plan. When that happens, it's tempting to blame the plan. But if you adhere to the plan God gives you, your success rate will be significantly better. Think about how you started this program and ask yourself if you have slacked off in any area. If so, list them here and then ask God to help you get back on track.

_____

_____

_____

_____

The Live It Plan was designed after much prayer by faithful followers of Christ. You are here because God brought you to this group, and He wants to work with you to bring your life into balance. Budgeting for balance will enable you to cooperate with Him to reach your goals. You might have to take some tough steps to adhere to the plan, but you can do it. Are you following your meal plan? Are you eating according to the amount of calories God has shown you to take in each day? Describe how you might work a little more closely with God in this area.

_____

_____

_____

Have you implemented some form of exercise into your weekly schedule? If so, describe it and the frequency. If not, take some time in prayer and write your exercise plan below.

_____

_____

_____

_____

The most important thing you can do to adhere to God's plan is to do *the next right thing*. What is the next right thing you should do today regarding your weight-loss efforts?

_____

_____

_____

_____

Jesus, I love it when a plan comes together. It's hard to visualize myself _____ pounds lighter right now; please help me get through the difficult days when I want to fall back into old habits. Amen.

Day 3 — CURB THE EXCESS

Father, I am willing to allow You to work in me so that I am better equipped to stop the excess in all areas of my life. I can't do it alone, Lord. Amen.

Have you shared with God your desire to start budgeting your activities, energy and talents in order to devote more time with Him? Have you expressed your intention to cooperate with God to lose the weight you

budgeting for balance | 47

need to lose for a healthier life? If so, you can move forward and take the next step in budgeting for balance: curbing the excess.

In managing your finances, identifying areas where you are over-spending is vital to reigning in your money. Problems such as not balancing your checkbook and failing to record all your checks and ATM withdrawals can result in devastating deficits, but financial advisors strongly suggest that a major problem in budget breakdowns comes from excessive spending, whether due to carrying too much cash or abusing credit cards. Curbing excess spending helps you stay within your budget.

Read Proverbs 21:5 and write a short description of how this verse provides guidance as you begin working on your life-in-balance budget.

_____

_____

_____

_____

Learning to live a balanced life means curbing the excess. In order to do that, you need to be diligent and rely on God's direction as you plan your meals. Take Joshua's advice in this week's memory verse to heart: "Be careful to obey all the law my servant Moses gave you; do not turn from it to the right or to the left, that you may be successful wherever you go." Circle any area(s) where you may have been overspending this week.

Mental   Physical   Spiritual   Emotional

Explain specifically how you have overspent and the effect it has had on your ability to live in balance.

_____

_____

_____

_____

_____

48 | week four

Whether you have spent too much effort worrying, being slothful, living according to the world's standards or indulging in unhealthy relationships, with God's help you can reign in your spending and live within a balanced life-budget. Read Matthew 11:28-30. What does this passage invite you to do with areas of your life where you are struggling?

_____

_____

_____

_____

_____

Use your prayer journal to unburden yourself to the Lord. Be specific about your concerns and give them to Jesus, asking Him to lighten your burden and provide rest for your soul.

Lord, You know the area of concern in my unbalanced life.
I need Your help to realign myself with Your plan for me. Show me
where to cut and change, and I will do my part each day to
curb the excess in my life. Amen.

Day 4

TRACKING EXPENSES IS VITAL

Lord, You are so faithful in how You care for me. Thank You
for helping me get this far and for forgiving me when I slip. Amen.

In First Place 4 Health, the Live It Tracker serves as your checkbook, tracking what you've spent on calories and revealing what you have left. Spending too many calories, especially empty ones, on junk food or foods that don't serve your body nutritionally will bankrupt your calorie account. The Live It Tracker serves as a budgeting tool when you make the time to learn how to use it, to maintain it and to evaluate it. Try recording your meals as you plan them instead of after you've eaten them; if you work in pencil, you can change your Tracker if your plans change.

budgeting for balance | 49

Read 1 Timothy 6:9-10. Think about when you overspend your calories. How does overspending cause you to fall into a trap and into many foolish and harmful desires?

_____

_____

_____

_____

Loving anything—including money and food—above God invites evil into our lives. How has your eagerness to satisfy your own desires pierced you "with many griefs" (see v. 10)?

_____

_____

_____

_____

How many days this week have you kept an accurate account of your calorie expenditures? Have you been spending excessively? If so, are you willing to focus on filling out your Live It Tracker the rest of this week? Carrying it with you throughout the day will make it more accessible. Using your calories wisely will help your body become healthier by providing fuel for you to serve the Lord with plenty of energy. Read Ephesians 5:15-17. In verse 15, what does Paul tell us to do?

_____

_____

_____

_____

In verse 17, what does Paul tell us _not_ to do?

_____

_____

_____

_____

week four

We are called to be good stewards of all that God has given to us. We are to manage everything God has entrusted to us, including our time, resources, money and calories. When we waste any of those, God will hold us accountable. Good stewards keep track of what they are managing.

God, forgive me for not managing things well. Help me to become a better steward of my calories, time and resources so that my life will be a reflection of You. Amen.

Day 5

BALANCED BUDGET PERKS

Thank You, Lord, for the peace that only You can give—a peace that comforts and loves, no matter what is going on around me. Amen.

Have you ever made a checkbook mistake and written a check for which your account did not have the funds? When this happens, the penalty fee is sometimes larger than the check amount! Invariably, you find out on a Friday afternoon and have to wait until Monday to reconcile the problem. It's upsetting—you're likely frustrated with yourself for not paying better attention to your checkbook and bank statement. The entire weekend—when you should be relaxing and preparing for the week ahead—you can't sleep, you have a headache and your stomach is upset.

On Monday you confront the bank (hoping that it was their mistake), only to discover that you entered a deposit twice. A lack of focused attention caused an error that resulted in a stressful weekend. From that experience, you learn that having things balanced has three perks that make your life more enjoyable and productive.

The first and best perk is *peace*. What does Paul say about our God in 1 Corinthians 14:33?

_____

_____

_____

_____

budgeting for balance | 51

Philippians 4:7 says, "The peace of God, which transcends all understanding, will guard your hearts and your minds in Christ Jesus." God is not a God of disorder, and when we allow any part of our life to fall into disarray—including our finances—we hinder our ability to be at our best for Him. A second perk of keeping things balanced is self-control. Read 1 Peter 5:8. What happens if we do not practice self-control?

When you relinquish control to Satan, he will take the opportunity to bring you down. He may tempt you with department store sales, trips or food. Credit card overuse is his specialty. When you are self-controlled and keep your checkbook balanced, Satan cannot load you up with guilt and anger. When you keep your finances in check, you will be blessed with confidence to manage your business. The last perk is *physical wellbeing*. A weekend of suffering with headaches, upset stomach and insomnia need not happen. When things get balanced on Monday, the headaches disappear, your stomach returns to normal and you sleep well. Read Proverbs 15:30. How does keeping things in balance contribute to a cheerful heart?

Making time to get things organized and balanced is worth pursuing. Feeling peaceful, self-controlled and physically fit contributes to the quality of our lives, allowing us to take the focus off of ourselves and become more loving and kind to others.

Lord, thank You for the lessons You teach me even through a bad checkbook experience; but more than that, thank You for Your mercy and grace. Amen.

52 | week four

Day
6

REFLECTION AND APPLICATION

Father, change is something I haven't handled well in the past.
I'm willing to listen and learn as You show me how to step outside my
comfort zone and adapt where necessary. Amen.

Reflect on what you have learned this week about budgeting—budgeting your finances and other areas of your life as well. If you spent quality time with God working on a plan to bring balance into your life, you may have been surprised by how He helped you change priorities. What surprised you the most when you and God sat down together to work through your activities—eliminating some, cutting back on others and maybe even adding different ones?

Change doesn't come easy for most people, so if you're having difficulty adapting, make it a matter of prayer. It may be a slow process, but everything God is teaching you through His Word is for your good. Read 2 Timothy 3:16-17. List the things verse 16 says Scripture is useful for.

What is the purpose of using Scripture in this way (v. 17)?

As you reflect on that passage, think about how God is using His Word to impact each area of your life. What are some specific Scripture verses or passages that are teaching, correcting, rebuking or training you mentally, physically, emotionally or spiritually? (For example, Matthew 6:33 may rebuke you regarding your spiritual priorities and challenge you to spend more time with God.)

Teaching

Rebuking

Correcting

Training in righteousness

Perhaps you have a story that you would like to share with your group about how God is using His Word in your life. Write about it here or in your journal. Don't forget to thank God for using His Word to help you budget for balance in your life.

_____

_____

_____

_____

_____

Father God, I am willing to do my part, and change is more than I can bear. I will ask for help from You and from those You have placed in my life. Amen.

Day 7

REFLECTION AND APPLICATION

Lord Jesus, as I reflect on this week, please show me what I need to focus on the most and teach me truths to apply to my life today. Amen.

Are you the type of person who welcomes structure or runs from it? Do you feel secure when you have a budget in place that guides you toward success, or do you feel stifled by it and prefer freedom? The Live It Plan is a structure that gives you freedom to choose from a myriad of delicious foods in all the food groups. Your Live It Tracker enables you to keep a record of your choices so that you know at a glance if you need to cut back.

Take a look at the Table of Contents of this Bible study, *Balanced Living*. What are some of the other First Place 4 Health resources in this book that can help you stay on track?

_____

_____

_____

_____

_____

budgeting for balance | 55

Which of the tools do you find the most helpful? Describe how they are working to make staying within your life-balance budget easier.

If there are one or more of these resources that you have not yet put to good use, are you willing to try one out in the week to come? Perhaps you can use the shopping lists and recipes, or track your miles for your daily walk or run. Pray about incorporating one or two of these tools into your life this week, and then write your commitment in the space below.

Tracking requires commitment and learning the basics requires effort. If you budget these things into your life, you *will* move closer to your goals. When you look at what you're spending and identify the leaks, you can fix them; but if you walk blindly, avoiding the problem and refusing to move outside your comfort zone, the help available from God does you no good. When you show up in the morning, meet with the Creator and acknowledge that it was *your* budgeting error that caused the problem, you will find peace, self-control and physical wellbeing!

Lord Jesus, please forgive me for ignoring the problem rather than dealing with what seems overwhelming to me. Help me learn to budget and make wise choices in each area of my life. Amen.

Group Prayer Requests

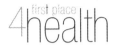

Today's Date: _____

Name	Request

Results

_____
_____
_____
_____

Week Five

CEO
secrets

SCRIPTURE MEMORY VERSE
*Therefore, prepare your minds for action;
be self-controlled; set your hope fully on the grace to be
given you when Jesus Christ is revealed.*
1 PETER 1:13

In the ever-changing financial world, a CEO may boast that his company is well-capitalized and has a strong balance sheet. He might feel that with solid investor backing and plenty of assets, his company is secure. He might spout words such as *healthy, solvent, intact* and *credible* to describe the soundness of his business. He has likely prepared himself with education, networking and hard work in order to make himself knowledgeable enough to build a profitable company. Yet even all of these financial, mental and educational assets do not change the fact that wealth can be fleeting; any sense of security he feels is, at the end of the day, false. Money cannot save him.

If you desire to achieve balance in your life, you would do well to prepare your mind for action and know what resources you have when hard times prevail—just like a good CEO. But the spiritual treasures of a Christian differ greatly from that of a CEO and can be trusted completely. A Christian's backing isn't stored in a bank vault or invested in stocks; nor are his assets measured by dollar signs. While a CEO may boast of his company's soundness, which is due to his own efforts, the Christian's secret is found in 1 Corinthians 1:31: "Therefore, as it is written: 'Let him who boasts boast in the Lord.' "

week five

Day 1

SPIRITUAL SOUNDNESS

Lord, as I begin this week hoping to discover secrets
that will help me be successful in my weight-loss journey,
help me prepare my mind for action and give me understanding. Amen.

How would you describe a sound business? Would it be one that is *solvent, reliable* and *tough*? There are many reasons people trust a company enough to buy its goods or hire its services, invest money in it, recommend it to others or go to work for it. You can check references, require financial statements and follow stock prices to get a good idea of a business's soundness. But what about a person's spiritual soundness—what are the earmarks that reveal to you his or her bottom line? How do you know your own spiritual soundness? God's Word provides sound principles that, if applied, will enable you to be sound and healthy in each area of your life.

Look up the following Scriptures and evaluate whether each description of spiritual soundness is present or absent in your life. (If one or more is absent, that is an area in which you have an opportunity to grow!)

Area	Scripture	Present	Absent
Stand firm	1 Cor. 15:58		
Continue in faith	Col. 1:22-23		
Faithful	1 Cor. 4:2		
Steadfast	Isa. 26:3		
Secure	Heb. 6:13-20		

CEO secrets | 59

Now look up the following passages in the first column, and then list the ways that Jesus performed the specific action indicated in the second column.

Scripture	Action	How Jesus performed this action
Matt. 27:11-14	Stood firm	
Luke 22:39-44	Continued in faith	
John 17:24-26	Showed Himself faithful	
John 18:19-24	Remained steadfast	
John 19:10-11	Knew He was secure	

Jesus says in John 10:28, "I give them eternal life, and they shall never perish; no one can snatch them out of my hand." Write a few sentences explaining how this verse helps you know that you are secure in Christ.

_____

_____

_____

_____

Jesus keeps you secure. Reading, studying and memorizing God's Word will give you the confidence you need to know you are not alone, not just in your weight-loss journey but in each area of your life, both in this life and the next. How secure do you feel about your eternal destination?

Unsure   I think I know   Fairly sure   Confident

What are the reasons you selected that option? What can you do to move to a deeper level of security in Christ?

_____

_____

_____

_____

Lord Jesus, having You in my heart, building a relationship with You and being able to call on You for help anytime gives me confidence that I can have victory and balance in all areas of my life. Amen.

Day 2 STAGNATE OR GROW

Father God, I do not want to stagnate and become dull. Show me through today's lesson how I can prevent that from happening. Amen.

CEOs generally keep a close eye on their balance sheets. The success of their businesses depends on their ability to stay abreast of trends and innovative ideas, as well as pay attention to the bottom line. They look to the advice of financial advisors to prevent their corporation from becoming stagnant. When a company begins to feel the pressures of a bad economy, its CEO must invest in new ideas that will help the company move forward, increase its vitality and turn a profit. Some companies may expand while others build on strengths and re-evaluate weaknesses. The one thing that a CEO cannot afford to do during tough economic times is nothing!

Stagnant means not moving or flowing, showing little or no sign of activity or advancement, or dullness from lack of change or development. Occasionally we get stuck "in a rut." When we're stuck, we may do repetitive things or say the same phrases over and over. Our routine rarely changes and we seem to be locked in the past rather than experiencing vitality and growth toward a promising future. Think about the words below that are aspects of stagnation and check which area(s) of your life is not moving or developing as it should.

	Mental	Physical	Spiritual	Emotional
Motionless				
Dull				
Sluggish				
Lacking vitality				
Unsuccessful				
Inactive				
Depressed				

Spend a few minutes thinking about the reasons that area(s) is impacted by stagnation. Why have you come to a standstill in that area of your life?

_____

_____

_____

_____

Look up the following Scriptures and describe how they might inspire your desire to get your life in balance.

Ezekiel 36:26

_____

_____

_____

week five

2 Corinthians 5:17

_____

_____

_____

Ephesians 4:24

_____

_____

_____

Like the CEO of a company, the one thing you cannot afford to do is nothing. Below, list one action in each area of your life that you are willing to take today in order to prevent stagnation or get things moving again. Then be prepared to share in your next group meeting what you did and what difference it made.

Mental

_____

_____

_____

_____

Physical

_____

_____

_____

_____

Spiritual

_____

_____

_____

_____

Emotional

_____

_____

_____

_____

Lord, having Your living water flowing through me means that I have Your power within me to change and grow. Help me begin to do that today. Amen.

CREDIBILITY IS KEY

Day 3

O my Lord, no one is more credible than You! My desire is to follow after You in all areas of my life. Amen.

Credibility doesn't happen overnight, but it is a key to staying competitive in business. A company must build its reputation for reliability by doing business in a trustworthy manner. It has great customer service, treats its customers with respect and guarantees its product or service. Great companies focus on building and maintaining credibility because it is much easier to retain satisfied customers than it is to recruit new ones, and once trust between customer and company is broken, it is almost impossible to get it back.

As Christians, we strive to be credible and bring glory to God in all areas of our life. We want to be a reflection of Jesus, and that means living in balance with Him at the center. The first part of this week's memory verse says, "Prepare your minds for action." Actions are important in developing credibility. What actions have you prepared in your mind to do this week that will help you be successful in First Place 4 Health? Circle all that apply (add your own if they are not listed).

Follow the Live It Plan   Exercise   Drink water

Pray   Memorize Scripture   Worship God

Other _____   _____   _____

Jesus Christ went to the cross and gave His life for you. He is trustworthy! He keeps His promises and gives unconditional love. Can He trust you to be honest and credible? To achieve success, it is important to be honest with yourself. Satan may try to deceive you, but the Holy Spirit within you is more powerful than Satan's lies. Be truthful with the Lord and He will give you victory!

Read Proverbs 12:22. What does the Lord detest?

What does He delight in?

Read Colossians 3:9-10. Who are we told not to lie to? Why?

Have you been honest concerning your efforts to lose weight since you began this program? Do your actions prove you credible? Does your walk match your talk? Use your journal to write a prayer to God concerning your credibility.

*Precious Lord, Your Word says that the truth will set me free
(see John 8:32). Help me always to speak the truth and let my actions
prove my credibility. Amen.*

WHERE YOUR TREASURES LIE

Day 4

Father, show me today the secret of storing up treasures in heaven for living the kind of life You want me to live. Amen.

Having a healthy bank account, a diverse stock portfolio and many material assets may seem like a solid foundation that will sustain you during a crisis. But wealth can dissipate quickly if the economy turns downward. Not only that, but also people who you trust with your money may prove themselves untrustworthy and deplete your investments, even in times of plenty.

The material possessions we own belong to God, and when we shift our focus off of Him and onto ourselves and our riches, we will inevitably be disappointed. God loves to bless His people with gifts, but when the gifts become more important than God, He is not pleased.

Where do your treasures lie? Today, we will look at several Scripture passages that can help us to understand how strongly God feels about this subject.

Read Deuteronomy 6:10-12. What did God promise to give to Israel when they reached the Promised Land?

_____

_____

_____

_____

_____

Was it fair that Israel would receive what others had worked for? (Read Genesis 12:1-9 for insight into this question, and keep in mind that the Promised Land was the same land God promised to Abraham.)

_____

_____

_____

_____

What is the warning given in Deuteronomy 6:12?

Read Matthew 6:19-20. In your own words, describe what happens to treasures stored up on earth.

In your own words, describe what happens to treasures that are stored up in heaven.

When we focus on material things, worrying that they may be destroyed or stolen, our attention and energy is taken away from God. We get out of balance when we strive to accumulate earthly possessions and forfeit heavenly treasures. List some practical ways that you can begin today storing up spiritual treasures.

Heavenly Father, there is nothing here on earth more important to me than You. I only need to look around and see Your handiwork to know that You are Creator of everything. Amen.

ASSETS AND RESOURCES

Day 5

Lord, help me to assess what I am investing in and what is most important to You. Show me where I need to make adjustments. Amen.

Each year the government publishes an "unclaimed money" list. People can check it to see if they have money due to them from an insurance policy, a land sale, a forgotten savings account or a relative's estate. If people do not claim it within a certain amount of time, the money reverts to the state.

Yesterday we learned that our treasures stored in heaven will never rust or decay and cannot be taken from us. Today we are going to learn how to claim spiritual treasures we may have overlooked.

One spiritual treasure you may not have considered is memorizing God's Word. So far in this study, we have had four memory verses to learn and put into action in our life. Can you recite all four? When you memorize them and apply each one to your life throughout the week, they help you to withstand the darts of the enemy.

Read Isaiah 55:10-11. In your own words, describe what is meant in verse 11 concerning the accomplishment of God's Word.

How does the principle of God accomplishing His purpose in your life through His Word help you feel confident and secure as you seek a life in balance?

week five

Prayer is a very important spiritual treasure because it is your direct link to God. Prayer provides direction, strength, peace, encouragement, vision and protection from the evil one. Read Philippians 4:6. What does it say we should do instead of feeling anxious? When should we do this?

_____

_____

_____

_____

Has the quality and quantity of your prayer time changed since you began this program? If so, how?

_____

_____

_____

_____

Another spiritual treasure is reading and studying God's Word. How can reading and studying Scripture be an asset to help you find balance in your life?

_____

_____

_____

_____

Acts 13:47 tells us that Paul and Barnabas were made a light for the Gentiles to bring salvation to the ends of the earth. Has the Lord made you a light for others? Describe a time when you were able to testify of God's work in your life. If you haven't yet had the chance, what would have to happen in your life in order for you to share your testimony?

_____

_____

_____

_____

Spiritual treasures are a Christian's resources for living a balanced life. When you begin storing them up and looking to God for help, you have all you need to reach your goals.

Father God, my spiritual bank account is filled with assets too numerous to list, and You send them to me at just the right time. Amen.

REFLECTION AND APPLICATION

Day
6

Lord, sometimes I feel motionless and unsuccessful. I think the effort of getting out of my rut is too difficult until I remember that nothing is too hard for You. Amen.

Healthy ponds contain moving water. When something prevents a pond's flow of water, problems occur. It can become a breeding ground for mosquitoes, algae and bacteria of all kinds and soon be an unsightly, unhealthy mess. Repairing the damage is much more time-consuming and expensive than preventing it, so it's wise to keep tabs on any body of water's influx and outflow of water. Look for clogs, seepage, erosion and other signs of stagnation and consult a professional for advice on repairs.

You learned this week some things about what stagnation looks like in a Christian's life. Just as with a pond, it's a good idea to inspect your life on a regular basis. You might want to spend a day with God to see if there is anything you need to unclog or repair. Is there some sin that needs to be confessed or habit that should be eliminated so living water can flow freely? Sin in one area can breed sin in other areas, throwing your life out of balance. Perhaps your life has become too busy, clogged up with unnecessary activities that erode your time with the Lord and bring your spiritual life to a standstill. Weakness due to inactivity may stagnate your physical strength and make you susceptible to illness. There may be people in your life who are like excessive algae in a pond. When pond algae exceed healthy limits, there are consequences: The oxygen level is reduced, the water turns cloudy and healthy plants and fish are suffocated. Sometimes relationships cause similar problems if they are not dealt with before they completely take over.

Today, reflect on what is happening in your life. Do you feel stuck, dull or motionless? Inspect the areas that you feel weakest in and ask God to show you how to repair what is out of balance so that you can move forward. This is a good project for your prayer journal or on a walk with God.

Dear Lord Jesus, You know my heart and my desire for balance and order, so I bring it all to You, the One who can change my life and move it toward health. Amen.

Day 7 REFLECTION AND APPLICATION

Lord, help me bring balance into my life. I need Your help to balance each area so that I'm walking upright on a firm foundation. Amen.

Think of your life as your "company" and yourself as its CEO. You want to be sure that you are spiritually sound and growing on a daily basis, because your company's health impacts all areas of your life and the lives of those close to you. Strangers can look at your company and be either drawn to God or pushed away from Him. In your journal or the spaces below, write your answers to the following questions.

How would you describe your "company" to someone who doesn't know the Lord? What words would you use and why? Look at your balance sheet and determine where you need to expand or strengthen. What actions will you take to avoid stagnation and get moving?

How does your company conduct business on a day-to-day basis? Can people look closely at your company and say that it is credible and trustworthy? How about God—what would He say? Can He trust you with His power? Is your company built soundly with Jesus Christ as the cornerstone? If not, are you willing to start fresh and ask Him to save your company from destruction?

Where are your treasures stored, here on earth or in heaven? Read Matthew 6:21 and then jot down some thoughts concerning your treasures. Make a list of your spiritual treasures and the earthly treasures that are most important to you. Which are more important?

Are your resources accessible? Review what spiritual assets you have available to get you through difficult times. List them according to which you will access first. How will making this list help you to balance your life in such a way that you will be successful in your weight-loss journey?

Lord God, when I let go and give You full control, I can move forward, growing and thriving. I set my hope fully on the grace You give. Amen.

Group Prayer Requests

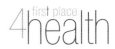

Today's Date: _____

Name	Request

Results

Week Six

possibilities and responsibilities

SCRIPTURE MEMORY VERSE

So give your servant a discerning heart to govern your people and to distinguish between right and wrong.

1 KINGS 3:9

If you could have absolutely anything in the world, what would it be? Wealth? Good health? Happiness? A beautiful home? Would you quit your job and travel around the world? Become a missionary? Would you isolate yourself in luxury or spend a fortune helping others?

A man featured in the newspaper some years ago won millions in the lottery. He quit his job and went on a spending spree. He began buying lavish big-boy toys, a new home and expensive furniture—and before a year had passed, he was broke. The man squandered his money, became an alcoholic and lost his wife and children. When he won his fortune, many possibilities lay before him, but he failed to realize that along with those possibilities came responsibilities.

Every day we wake up to endless possibilities for how to spend our time, money, energy and thoughts. We are responsible for using them for our and others' good and to ensure that they are pleasing to God. Everything we have comes from and belongs to God. He blesses us richly in all things—so long as we put His kingdom, interests and principles first in our lives. When we seek God, He blesses us with what we need and so much more. We must always remember to use wisely the blessings He sends our way.

week six

Day 1

BE CAREFUL WHAT YOU ASK FOR

Heavenly Father, give me discernment in how to use Your gifts in ways that bring joy to others and glory to You. Amen.

Sarah and Doug attended an open house in a very elite section of town. One 3,600 square foot, two-story home combined the charm of the old with the luxury of the new. Filled with innovative ideas, architecture, art and design, it included three bedrooms, three-and-a-half bathrooms, home office, gourmet kitchen and two-car garage. Outside, the house welcomed visitors with front and back porches and a landscape designed with outdoor entertaining in mind. They put in an offer and eagerly waited for the phone call telling them that the dream home was theirs.

The day came and they moved in, believing that God had blessed them. Two years later, Doug lost his executive job with a land development company because of bad judgment higher up—just as Sarah discovered that she was pregnant. Money problems hit and they fell behind in the enormous mortgage payments. They began arguing and went to their pastor for counseling.

In the end, they realized that they had convinced themselves that God wanted them to have the house. Doug and Sarah did what many people do: They made their decision and moved ahead before waiting on the Lord. Now they advise, "Be careful what you ask for . . . you might get it!"

Do you have something in your heart today that you earnestly long to have? Take a moment and write your heart's desire here or in your journal. Make it a prayer and tell God what it means to you.

_____

_____

_____

_____

_____

possibilities and responsibilities | 75

Once you have shared your desire with God, it is time to wait on Him. Are you willing to wait patiently and accept God's decision? Patience is a character trait God longs to cultivate in each of His people. Many times, He delays blessings until we are mature enough to handle them responsibly. He knows and provides for our needs, and at the proper time in His plan for us He will send blessings as well. The answer may not be exactly as we hope for, but it will be for our good.

In your own words, what does Matthew 6:33 say?

_____

_____

_____

_____

This week's memory verse records King Solomon's request to God. Instead of riches and glory in battle, Solomon asked for wisdom. Read 1 Kings 3:9-14. Did God grant Solomon's request? What else did God provide for him?

_____

_____

_____

_____

Read 1 Kings 11:1-10. Do you think that Solomon responsibly used the wisdom that God gave him? Why or why not?

_____

_____

_____

_____

Solomon was a wise king throughout his rule but failed to act wisely in his own household. He began by going against God's command by marrying the pharaoh's daughter. He taxed and worked his people excessively, eventually alienating them. Solomon began by laying a foundation with God, but did not follow through later in life. Have you started with God and somewhere along the way lost your balance? How did it happen?

What or who are you allowing to lead you: fleshly desires or the Holy Spirit? In what ways?

God, I need and depend on You for wisdom. Help me know
what to do and give me the power to do it. Amen.

Day 2 — ONE SERVANT'S MOTIVE

Search me O God, and know my heart; test me and know my
anxious thoughts. See if there is any offensive way in me,
and lead me in the way everlasting (Psalm 139:22-24). Amen.

The word "servant" has taken on negative connotations in our culture. Many people associate it with slavery, mindless obedience or degrading employment. Then there are those called "public servants," whose motives range from a hunger for power, a love of country or a desire for change. Sometimes it is unclear whether they are servants of the public or of their own ambitions.

Christians, however, recognize that being a servant is the highest order of achievement. God's servants relinquish personal motives and achievements and welcome His will for their lives. They are motivated by the love of a compassionate God.

possibilities and responsibilities | 77

Read Philippians 2:5-8 and describe what your attitude should be like.

In verse 7, what nature did Jesus take on?

Do you consider yourself a servant of God? Write down an area of your life in which you are serving Him, along with your motives for doing so. Be honest as you search your heart.

Do you think God is pleased with your motives? Give specific reasons for your answer.

Reread this week's memory verse, paying attention to Solomon's desire and how he regarded his role. How did he view himself?

Solomon loved the Lord and considered himself God's servant. He also knew that to do the job he was called to do—governing Israel with wisdom and justice—he needed God's help. He expressed his desire in

week six

1 Kings 3:9, the first part of which is this week's memory verse: "So give your servant a discerning heart to govern your people and to distinguish between right and wrong. For who is able to govern this great people of yours?" The last part of the verse is a rhetorical question, but it reveals something about Solomon's motives. Do you think God was convinced of Solomon's motives for asking for wisdom? Why or why not?

_____

_____

_____

_____

God saw that Solomon wanted to use wisdom to govern His people. He gave Solomon much more than he asked for because Solomon, a servant of God, had the right motive. What is your motive for being in First Place 4 Health? Be honest and search your heart, asking the Holy Spirit to reveal to you what is hidden there.

_____

_____

_____

_____

Heavenly Father, I want to share with others Your unfailing love and mercy. Give Your servant wisdom and discernment to make wise decisions. Amen.

Day 3

A DISCERNING HEART

Lord, grant me understanding and insight. Teach me the right things to do and shine brightly through me for others to see. Amen.

We have all seen commercials or cartoons that feature a character with a red-horned devil perched on one shoulder and a cute little angel on the other. They take turns whispering in the character's ears, one tempting her to do wrong and the other guiding her with heavenly direction. Occasionally the little devil wins, tempting the individual with chocolate to please her palate or sex to satisfy her fleshly desires. But the angel combats each temptation with wisdom and discernment, anticipating the devil's next attempt to lead the person astray.

As you make progress on your weight-loss journey, you will be tempted to make poor decisions. Why? Because of Satan. He wants you to fail so that others will discredit God. We may laugh at the idea of a red-horned devil perched on our shoulder, but it is a fact that Satan prowls around, trying to prevent God's people from doing the right thing (see 1 Peter 5:8). He cannot take a Christian's soul, but he can devour their testimony and try to prevent them from leading others to know the Lord. The Holy Spirit within us whispers wisdom and will give us a discerning heart; if we follow His leading, we will not be led astray.

Read 1 Kings 3:16-28. In your words, explain the case that was brought before King Solomon.

_____

_____

_____

_____

Describe the method King Solomon used to discern who the real mother was (vv. 24-25).

_____

_____

_____

_____

What prompted Solomon to use this method to reveal the child's mother? Did he know what the outcome would be? Why or why not?

_____

_____

_____

_____

When Israel heard the verdict the king had given, they were in awe (v. 28). Why?

_____

_____

_____

_____

How do you think wisdom and discernment from the Holy Spirit can help you on your First Place 4 Health journey?

_____

_____

_____

_____

God, when I ask with the right motive, You generously give me what I need.
Help me remember to always look to You for help. Amen.

Day 4 — RECOGNIZING TRUTH

Jesus, You are my compass for living a balanced life. Keep me going
in the right direction so my life will stay on course. You are
my Way, my Truth and my Life (John 14:6). Amen.

When the Treasury Department trains people to spot forgeries, they focus on studying *real* bills, not fakes. They learn every detail, mark and color of genuine bills so that they can tell at a glance when they are looking at a fake. They do not study the forgery to know the truth!

There are many false prophets out there clamoring to pull unsuspecting people away from the truth and lead them to hell. Satan specializes in deception and will never stop his lies (see John 8:44). But it's silly to think that by studying Satan we can detect his lies; instead, we must study the truth in God's Word. That way, we will know the truth and the truth will set us free.

possibilities and responsibilities | 81

Read Hebrews 6:13-18 and fill in the missing words from verse 18.

God did this so that, by _____ _____
_____ in which it is _____ for God to
_____, we who have fled to take hold of the _____ offered
to us may be greatly _____.

God's nature is unchangeable and He cannot lie. He kept His promise and oath to Abraham and continues to do the same for us. Read Isaiah 45:19. What does the Lord speak? What does He declare?

_____

_____

_____

_____

Hebrews 13:8 says, "Jesus Christ is the same yesterday and today and forever." Knowing this will enable you to discern what is right and recognize truth. Satan will not be able to deceive and destroy you when you stand firm and resist him with the unchanging truth of our Lord. How has reading God's Word helped you to stand firm when you have been tempted?

_____

_____

_____

_____

Have you used the First Place 4 Health memory verses to resist Satan? Explain how.

_____

_____

_____

_____

_____

Today, commit to spending quality time reading Scripture each day and memorizing it. The more you are in His Word, the more you will know Him intimately, be able to discern between right and wrong, recognize false prophets and see through Satan's lies.

*My Lord Jesus, I love discovering everything about You
and learning what You have for me each day. Teach me Your ways
so that I can discern between right and wrong. Amen.*

Day 5 — REJECTING WRONG

*Father, You are supreme over all things and I am under the protection of
Your wings. Thank You for covering me with Your love. Amen.*

Think about the words "reject" and "eject." Picture a fighter jet soaring through the air when suddenly something goes wrong. The pilot does all he can to set things right, but if he is unable to fix the problem before a crash, he must reject the temptation to stay too long; he pulls the "Eject" lever to save his life. In an instant, he is expelled from the aircraft and his parachute is deployed.

Read Genesis 19:15-25. What did the angels instruct Lot to do? Why?

_____

_____

_____

_____

In your own words, what was Lot's reply (v. 19)?

_____

_____

_____

_____

_____

possibilities and responsibilities | 83

Lot's life was at stake. God was about to destroy the city of Sodom and everyone in it because of the evil perpetrated there. But instead of pulling that "Eject" lever, he negotiated with the angels, begging them to allow him to go to a small town named Zoar. Read verses 24-25 and describe in your own words what the Lord did.

_____

_____

_____

_____

Look at verse 17. What did the angels instruct Lot and his family *not* to do?

_____

_____

_____

_____

What does verse 26 tell us happened to Lot's wife?

_____

_____

_____

_____

When we are tempted to indulge in wrong—whether it is eating poorly, addictions, immorality or idolatry—ejecting ourselves can save our lives. Doing what the world thinks is right is often wrong in God's eyes. He wants us to *reject* wrong and *eject* ourselves from the tempting situation. We are not to follow the crowd, but to use wisdom from God to make choices for our good. Describe a recent situation when you needed to reject the wrong and eject yourself. Be specific.

_____

_____

_____

_____

How did you handle it? Did you eject yourself or stay around to suffer the consequences?

_____

_____

_____

_____

One important way that you can flee and not conform to the pattern of the world is by allowing God to transform you by renewing your mind. Read Romans 12:2. What will you be able to do if your mind is renewed?

_____

_____

_____

_____

Read and meditate on Genesis 19:29. God remembered Abraham and rescued Lot, and He will keep His promise to you as well. Don't look back. Keep your eyes on the Savior.

> *God, help me reject wrong when I find myself in its midst*
> *by ejecting immediately. Transform me, Lord, by renewing my mind.*
> *Give me Your thoughts and help me to focus on You. Amen.*

Day 6

REFLECTION AND APPLICATION

Show me the truth You have for me today, Lord. Help me
understand the importance of distinguishing between right and wrong
and to choose right—quickly. Amen.

Most parents know when their children are not being truthful. They recognize certain body language and mannerisms—the rolling eyes, shoulder shrugs and fast breathing are a dead giveaway. Many parents know their kids are lying even when they talk to them on the telephone and

possibilities and responsibilities | 85

can't see their face. There is something in their voice, a nervous tone or a hesitant answer, that gives them away.

Do you think God knows when His children are not being truthful with Him? Of course He does. Adam tried hiding from God in the garden, but it didn't work; God knew exactly where Adam was and what he was doing. He also knows the deepest crevice of your heart and the secret motives and untruths that you may not even have admitted to yourself. The great news is that He will give you many opportunities to confess.

Read Proverbs 6:16-19. Write in your own words what the Lord hates.

_____

_____

_____

_____

Read the story of Ananias and Sapphira in Acts 5:1-11. What did Ananias and Sapphira lie about?

_____

_____

_____

_____

In your own words, what did Peter say to Ananias in verses 3-4?

_____

_____

_____

_____

Who did Peter say Ananias and Sapphira were lying to?

_____

_____

_____

_____

86 | week six

Think about this story in relation to your First Place 4 Health journey. Have you tried to deceive God in any way? In your journal or the space below, confess to Him any instance when you have told less than the complete truth. Spend time with the Lord and ask forgiveness. He's waiting.

_____

_____

_____

_____

Lord God, help me to come to You and confess my dishonesty and
give me strength to resist Satan's attempts to destroy my testimony. Amen.

Day 7

REFLECTION AND APPLICATION

Lord, teach me Your ways and guide my feet along Your path.
Help me reflect on You and recognize Your voice at every turn. Amen.

In the book of Proverbs, we are given wise sayings and good advice. Proverbs 1:8-19 contains four "do nots" for all who are seeking wisdom both spiritually and practically. What are they?

Do not _____ _____ _____ _____ (v. 8).

Do not _____ _____ (v. 10).

Do not _____ _____ _____ _____ (v. 15).

Do not _____ _____ _____ _____ _____ (v. 15).

Think about the people in your life. Do any of them entice you to make poor choices in any of the four areas of your life? Describe a specific situation you are dealing with right now, and how the four "do nots" listed above can help you stay on track.

_____

_____

_____

_____

possibilities and responsibilities | 87

Look up the proverb that corresponds with today's date and read through it. (For example, if today is October 10, read Proverbs 10.) Ask God to give you wisdom to help you with the situation you described above. In your journal or below, record what God reveals to you in your reading today.

The poetry of the psalms and the wisdom of the proverbs reflect the high value ancient Hebrews placed on skillful craftsmanship. The poets, musicians and philosophers crafted these Old Testament books with excellence, to pay God the honor due to Him. Today, we can honor God with our minds, bodies, hearts and spirits using the tools He has provided. What will you do today to honor Him?

There are 31 proverbs—the perfect number to read one every day of the month. Ask the Holy Spirit to reveal a new truth each day as you read the corresponding day's chapter. Then write in your journal how you will apply it to your life.

Father in heaven, help me keep my eyes on You instead of following others who would entrap me and cause me to fail. Today, Lord, teach me Your truth and show me how I can make it real in my life. Amen.

Group Prayer Requests

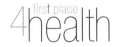

Today's Date: _____

Name	Request

Results

Week Seven

lawful or helpful

SCRIPTURE MEMORY VERSE
*"Everything is permissible for me"—but not everything is beneficial.
"Everything is permissible for me"—but I will not be mastered by anything.*
1 CORINTHIANS 6:12

Just because something is legal doesn't always make it right. For example, in the United States, people of a certain age are able to purchase cigarettes and alcohol. Many people live together outside of marriage, and hundreds of thousands of teen (and some preteen) girls become pregnant each year. Sexually transmitted diseases are on the rise, and divorce now claims half of all marriages.

In Paul's day, the people of Corinth lived in a city where many immoral activities were legal (and, in some cases, even encouraged), and the new Christians weren't sure what behaviors were okay and which ones weren't. Some of the things they were doing were not acceptable for God's children. In his letters, Paul tried to help the Corinthian church understand that freedom should be used to glorify God and help others—not to indulge self.

This week we will explore our own permissive actions as it relates to our health, and seek out ways to wisely use the freedom that Jesus provided; we will come to understand that we are free *from* sin, not free *to* sin. There is a big difference in the two words *permissible* and *permissiveness*. What separates the two is choice. You are given the opportunity, as a Christian freed from the law and placed under grace, to make choices that affect your entire life. God offers His help and guidance, but you can choose not to trust and obey what He tells you.

Before you began your journey toward whole-life balance with First Place 4 Health, what out-of-balance diets did you try? Think about how those choices affected your body. They may have worked initially, but they also may have damaged your metabolism, self-image and motivation. Can you honestly say that you were "free"? Giving God permission to help you balance your life is the best choice—the choice that affirms your freedom in Christ. He's waiting to show you what real freedom means and how to use it wisely.

Day 1 — FREEDOM GRANTED

Thank You, Lord, for freeing me from sin so that I can live eternally with You. Show me how to live out that freedom in a way that honors You. Amen.

An "exodus" is an exit or a departure. One of the best examples of God caring for His people is found in the Old Testament book of Exodus. God granted the Israelites their freedom from Egyptian slavery and oppression. God Himself guided them toward the Promised Land in a pillar of cloud by day and a pillar of fire by night. They were finally free! The story of the Israelites includes some harrowing challenges, a few shameful sins and many restored lives. God granted them freedom, but, as often happens today, they misused and abused their freedom. The Israelites rebelled, set up idols, complained and continued in sin.

Read Exodus 16:1-3. Shortly after the Israelites left Egypt, they began complaining. Look closely at verse 3: "The Israelites said to them, 'If only we had died by the Lord's hand in Egypt! There we sat around pots of meat and ate all the food we wanted, but you have brought us out into the desert to starve this entire assembly to death.'" They would rather have died in bondage with all the food they could eat than to live in freedom and experience physical hunger pains! They seem to have forgotten what their enslavement in Egypt was really like.

lawful or helpful | 91

Can you look back to the time before you asked God to help you with your weight and remember eating whatever you wanted? Did you feel that you had the freedom to eat anything you wanted regardless of its effect on your body? Have you complained about the smaller portions that you are eating now? How has your attitude been similar to that of the Israelites?

Describe the difference between freedom *to* overeat and freedom *from* overeating.

Read John 8:31-36. After reading verse 36, fill in the blanks:

So if the _____ sets you _____, you will be _____ indeed.

Who sets you free and what are you set free from?

In verse 31 Jesus told the Jews, "If you hold to my teaching you really are my disciples." In the Greek, the word for hold is *meno*, which means to continue, remain, abide or dwell. Considering this meaning, give some examples of how you are holding to His teachings as you go through this session of First Place 4 Health.

_____

_____

_____

_____

Read the following Scripture passages and describe what it says about God in each.

Psalm 18:2

_____

_____

_____

_____

Psalm 18:30-31

_____

_____

_____

_____

Psalm 46:1

_____

_____

_____

_____

Psalm 91:2

_____

_____

_____

_____

After reading those assurances, what specific action will you take to trust God's plan for your freedom?

My God, please help me to live in the freedom You provided on the cross, to walk upright and to stand firm in the face of trouble. Amen.

THE CHOICE IS YOURS

Day 2

Lord, I want to be a reflection of You from the time I get up until I lay my head down at night. Help me sort through all that is before me. Amen.

Our culture has an "If it feels good, do it" mentality, and sometimes it is hard to distinguish between what behaviors are acceptable in the eyes of God and what behaviors are culturally permitted just because we are adults. God's Word is specific about many things, yet some difficult choices seem to be in a gray area.

Read Hebrews 5:13-14. What kind of person lives on milk? Who takes in solid food? Explain the difference.

Regarding where you are in your weight-loss journey, what type of spiritual food are you taking in—milk or solids?

Those of us who are new to First Place 4 Health must learn the basics of the Live It Plan and what it means to live with Christ in the center of our life; these simple disciplines are the "milk" that strengthens us for future maturity. There is no "gray area" when it comes to the basics. Yet as we grow and mature, making Bible study, prayer and Christian fellowship into "solid" habits, we will encounter more and more areas of life that are not all black and white. When that happens, we can trust the Holy Spirit to guide and direct us as we seek God's heart.

You can discover how God feels about a few "gray areas" by reading His Word. Look up the following Scriptures and write down in your own words what you discover about God's view of each topic.

Scripture	Topic	God's view
2 Cor. 9:7	Giving	
Matt. 6:28-30	Worry	
Matt. 6:14	Forgiveness	

The more time you spend reading Scripture and meditating on it, the better you will become familiar with how God wants you to live. God cares about every aspect of our lives. When you know how He feels about something, it is easier to make the choice that will bring balance into your life. The choice is yours: to use your freedom to glorify God or to live for yourself.

lawful or helpful | 95

Read Galatians 6:7-9. What is the "meat" of this verse, in your own words?

_____

_____

_____

_____

Father God, I want to spend more time building our relationship
and understanding Your heart. Help me to avoid the permissiveness
in today's world by standing strong and doing right. Amen.

STUMBLING BLOCK

Day
3

Lord, show me today if I am a stumbling block in anyone's life,
and help me daily to live a life pleasing to You. Amen.

Christians sometimes use the word "freedom" as an excuse to continue dabbling in things of the world, claiming that they are no longer under the law. While our salvation *is* a free gift of God and is not determined by our following a set of laws, attempts to work off sin or being legalistic, we must take great care that our actions don't send mixed signals to a new Christian or someone struggling in their Christian life. If we cause them to stumble into sin due to our example, we will have to answer to God for it.

Building up the faith of a sister or brother in Christ should take priority over our freedom to do this or that. We may not be aware, but others are watching and often imitating our actions. If we continuously strive to imitate Christ, then we need not fear having someone follow what we do and how we live.

Read Romans 14:13-23. How are we to prevent becoming a stumbling block (v. 13)?

_____

_____

_____

_____

How can you know when something you are doing may be a stumbling block for someone else?

_____

_____

_____

_____

Read verse 15 again, and then fill in the blanks below:

If your brother is distressed because of what you eat, you are _____

_____ _____ _____ _____ .

Describe an activity that is permissible for you that was or has the potential to be a stumbling block to a brother or sister in Christ. Alternatively, describe an activity that is permissible for a brother or sister in Christ that has been or is a stumbling block for you. (You may write about this in your journal if you are concerned about privacy.)

_____

_____

_____

_____

_____

God is working in each of us in a unique way. If you listen to God, He will reveal what is permissible for you. Sometimes, however, even though you have the freedom to do certain activities, you may be free to do it only in private. Write verse 22 in your own words as if you were recording a conversation between you and God.

_____

_____

_____

_____

_____

Read verses 19-21 again and ask God to help you live out your freedom in a way that will not cause others to stumble.

My God, help me discern when, where and how to use the freedom You so generously provided. Remind me not to judge how others live out their own freedom. Amen.

FOLLOW THE MASTER

Day
4

Help me, Lord, to stay on the path You have laid out for me. When I veer from it, cause me to return and keep my eyes focused on You. Amen.

Have you ever wondered whether what you are hearing is really coming from God? In order to live a balanced life, we need to follow after our Lord. When we follow Him, we will be able to discern between what will or will not be beneficial to us. Scripture tells us that we can know His voice and identify it from all possible sources of deception.

In John 10:3-5, Jesus provides us with an example of the instinctive nature of sheep: They listen to the voice of their shepherd and recognize him. In the same way, we too can discern between God's voice if we come to know His character, nature and how He acted in the lives of those who have gone before us. Read Malachi 3:6 and Numbers 23:19. How do these passages describe God's character?

_____

_____

_____

_____

The fact that God does not change or lie helps us identify whether what we are hearing is actually coming from Him, because when He speaks, He never contradicts what is in His Word. His voice will give us wisdom and common sense to do what is right. During this study, what are some things the Lord has spoken to you that you knew were from Him rather than from a deceptive source? How did you discern they were from Him?

Have you ever heard anything in your spirit that you felt was not from God? If so, explain what it was and how you discerned that it was not from Him.

Read Hebrews 4:12. How does the author describe God's Word?

We have God's authoritative Word, and through it we are able to cut through the deceptions of the enemy that threaten to take us off course. What are some ways that you can better enable God's Word to flow through your life and help you to discern and obey the Lord's voice?

Lord Jesus, my Shepherd, my Master and Savior, help me to always recognize Your voice and follow after You. Amen.

lawful or helpful | 99

LED BY THE SPIRIT

Day 5

*Jesus, forgive me when I allow food or habits to control me
and cause me to lose sight of my goals. Help me today to remember that
You are my Master and that I am led by Your Holy Spirit. Amen.*

We are saved by God's grace, but we still experience fleshly desires. When the flesh controls us, the flesh wins; but if we allow the Holy Spirit living within us to lead, we can be free of the flesh's control. He provides us with power to resist temptation and Satan's schemes for knocking us down when we least expect it.

Read Galatians 5:16-18. We are told in verse 16 to live by the Spirit. What does it tell us will be the result of doing so?

_____

_____

_____

_____

The phrase "live by" implies *surrendering to* or *being encompassed/embraced by* in the original Greek. We are to surrender to the Holy Spirit's embrace. What are some specific ways that you can do that as you participate in the First Place 4 Health program?

_____

_____

_____

_____

Galatians 5:19-21 list acts of the sinful nature. Write down any that might be hazardous to your health (mental, physical, spiritual or emotional).

_____

_____

_____

_____

100 | week seven

What does Paul say in verse 21 about those who live by the sinful nature?

_____

_____

_____

_____

Verses 22-23 list characteristics of those who live by the Spirit. Pick any three "fruit" and describe how they can have a positive impact on your health (mental, physical, spiritual or emotional).

_____

_____

_____

_____

_____

Read verse 24. Who has crucified the sinful nature with its passions and desires?

_____

_____

_____

_____

Verse 25 tells us how we can live as those who belong to Christ Jesus:

Since we _____ by the _____, let us _____
____ _____ with the _____.

Our sinful nature and fleshly desires are in a battle against the Holy Spirit who lives within us. Only with the power and strength of Jesus Christ, who won our freedom for His glory, can we resist doing unhealthy and sinful things lurking in the shadows. We must choose daily to surrender to and be embraced by the Spirit. When we do that, God's power overcomes the flesh—and we will find victory.

*Thank You, Jesus, for sending Your Holy Spirit, who enables me
to fight fleshly desires and passions that want to defeat me.
I want to be a place of peace where Your Holy Spirit can reside. Amen.*

REFLECTION AND APPLICATION

Day
6

*Father, help me see what You want me to apply to my life.
Give me wisdom and strength as I listen for Your voice. Amen.*

On Day 4 this week, we learned about following the Master by knowing
His voice. In thinking about voices you may have followed before you
came into First Place 4 Health, describe how they led you down a path
of deception, particularly where your body is concerned. List as many as
you can remember and take time to reflect on how you felt when you realized that what you were doing was just not working.

_____

_____

_____

_____

Think now about hearing how God speaks to you through His Word.
How does it help you to live a more balanced life? Name some examples
of choosing not to do some things that, while they are permissible, are
not beneficial to you right now.

_____

_____

_____

_____

Jesus is a Good Shepherd who cares deeply for each of His children, His
sheep. A shepherd leads his flock with faithfulness, compassion, guidance
and protection. How has the Lord shown those characteristics to you?
Spend some time praising Him today for His faithful and compassionate

guidance and protection. Write a prayer of thankfulness below or in your journal for your freedom from the many masters who once held you in bondage.

Oh Lord, I am so thankful that I will never have to be enslaved again.
You redeemed me and paid for all of my sins—past, present and future.
You are my hope and I gladly follow You wherever You take me. Amen.

Day 7 · REFLECTION AND APPLICATION

Beautiful Savior, I praise Your name and sing songs of joy
because of all You have done for me. Thank You for
the song in my heart as I serve You. Amen.

Today, think about the difference between things that are both permissible *and* beneficial and actions that are permissible but *are not* beneficial. Make a list below of some foods, activities (physical, social, hobbies, and so on) or relationships that are both permissible and beneficial.

Permissible	Beneficial

lawful or helpful | 103

Now make a list of foods, activities or relationships that are permissible but are not beneficial. These are not "bad" foods, activities or relationships, but they may cause you to lose sight of your goals or to become a stumbling block for others.

Permissible	Reason not beneficial

Write this week's memory verse (from memory!) in the space below.

Take time to pray about the things you listed that are not beneficial for you right now. Ask God to help you relinquish your hold on them. If it's a certain food, activity or hobby, you may need to set it aside for a season. If a relationship is an issue, perhaps God has a better plan for it. Be honest with God about your feelings and allow Him to change your attitude and focus.

Lord and Savior, I know that some things are not really beneficial for me.
They may even cause me to be a stumbling block for someone else.
I want to choose things that will glorify You and edify me. Amen.

Group Prayer Requests

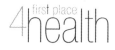

Today's Date: _____

Name	Request

Results

Week Eight

designed by the master

SCRIPTURE MEMORY VERSE
Unless the LORD builds the house, its builders labor in vain.
PSALM 127:1

The great American architect Frank Lloyd Wright (1867-1959) had his own philosophy about designing homes. He balanced the needs of owners with the particular qualities of the location of the home. In 1991, he was named "the greatest American architect of all time" by the American Institute of Architects,[1] and his work is still admired by many. He understood the importance of bringing balance into every home he built, and making each design unique.

Our Master Builder, Jesus Christ, understands every detail of what goes into building a house, and He knows how to balance each area of our mental, emotional, physical and spiritual life. We are individually unique; no two are alike. He knows our deepest needs because He designed our particular qualities.

Our life is a work in progress as we journey through the years, and the Master balances out what we allow to shift or run down. Often we attempt to remodel the original design only to discover that we have used faulty materials, left out important details or created too much busyness. When that happens, we have to go back to the drawing board and begin again. If we have left the Master out of our plans, our life will be out of plumb and we will be unbalanced in one or more areas. We may choose defective materials and trust them to last, or choose quantity over quality and suffer the consequences. When we leave Him out and build on our own, it will all be done in vain. But when we study God's Word and allow Him to design and build our life, it will be a place of functional beauty that will last.

Day 1 CHILDHOOD TALE

Master Jesus, show me how to build a life that will be glorifying to You, fit for a child of the King! Amen.

We are all familiar with the story of those three pigs and how each of them designed and built what they thought was the perfect house. The first pig used straw, the second used sticks and the third built his abode with bricks. The Big Bad Wolf blew down the first two pigs' houses, while the wise third pig lived in safety and comfort in his solid, sturdy brick house.

Jesus told a similar parable about building. Read Matthew 7:24-27. What does Jesus say the wise man built his house on?

_____

_____

_____

_____

If we want to build our lives on the Rock, what are two things that we must do (v. 24)?

1. _____

2. _____

Describe what happens when we do those two things (v. 25).

_____

_____

_____

designed by the master | 107

Read verses 26-27, and describe what kind of person hears the words but doesn't put them into practice. What happens to the house he has built?

_____

_____

_____

_____

In First Place 4 Health, you engage in daily Bible study. In this way, you "hear" Jesus' words. What are some specific ways that you put His words into practice?

_____

_____

_____

_____

Verse 25 contains an important message for how to build your house. Read it again and then fill in the blanks.

Yet it did not fall, because it had its _____

on the _____.

Jesus is sometimes called "the Rock," a word-picture drawn from the book of Psalms. When we begin building or rebuilding with Jesus Christ, from the ground up, He becomes our foundation. He prevents our life from becoming unbalanced and toppling over. He is our strength during life's storms, and our anchor when we are hit by the winds of change. Describe one specific way that having Jesus as your foundation has brought more balance and stability to your life.

_____

_____

_____

_____

Think back to the story of the Three Little Pigs. In some versions of the story, when the Big Bad Wolf came to the door, the first little pig got frightened and ran away squealing. The second one disappeared, never to be seen again. And the third? The wisest little pig had confidence in the strength of his structure and outwitted the enemy. Which most represents you when it comes to First Place 4 Health? Why?

_____

_____

_____

_____

Dear Jesus, my Rock, thank You for the confidence that comes with knowing You are there to protect and shelter me when the wolf knocks on my door. Amen.

Day 2 — CHOOSING MATERIALS

Lord, please help me to choose wisely what materials to use to build my life. Show me what will last so that I have a goal to work toward. Amen.

Some contractors are so concerned with building a project cheaply that they cut corners by using inferior materials. This practice usually catches up with them, however, when home inspectors uncover their shoddy business practices. When that happens, the contractors are fined and must pay for the fixes; cheating their customers ends up costing them much more in the long run than if they had chosen quality materials from the start.

Even when inspections fail to expose the use of poor materials, the truth always comes out. One such case involved a house that caught fire. The home was destroyed, along with the family's car and beloved pets, and the flames threatened a neighbor's house as well. During the subsequent investigation, faulty wiring that had not been installed correctly was discovered to be the cause of the fire. The electrical contractor was

designed by the master | 109

financially liable for the damages. In an effort to increase his profit, he used cheap materials that led to the destruction of property, animals and his reputation.

Read 1 Corinthians 3:10-15. What is the warning given in the last part of verse 10?

What does Paul say in verses 13-14 about the quality of the materials a person uses when building on the foundation laid by Christ?

Is the foundation of your life built on Jesus Christ? If so, describe how that foundation was laid. If you're not sure, write a short prayer asking Jesus to be your foundation. (If you need help, your leader will be happy to guide you.)

The materials you have been using to build on your foundation since you began First Place 4 Health include prayer, daily Scripture reading, Scripture memorization, exercise, following the Live It plan and group participation. Think about how you are using these materials. Are you memorizing a verse to say at weigh in and then forgetting it later, or are you using it to guard your heart against temptation? Are you making the Live It into a diet to try losing weight faster, or are you following it to become healthy and fit? Describe how practices like these could end up costing you more in the long run.

_____

_____

_____

_____

Read Revelation 4:10-11 and meditate on it. What are you building in this life that will honor your Lord in the next?

_____

_____

_____

_____

You are worthy, my Lord, to receive glory and honor and power.
It is by Your will that I was created, and I thank You. Amen.

Day 3

LABOR IN VAIN

Help me, God, to not labor in vain, but to make each day count
for Christ as I see Your design for me being carried out. Amen.

Every summer, thousands of people head to the beach to view beautiful sand castles and sculptures that professional and amateur artists have labored untold hours to build. They use specialized tools to create their masterpieces and compete in contests around the world for prizes ranging from blue ribbons to greenbacks. They receive recognition from their peers for their works of art and provide entertainment for the masses.

But what happens in the end? Are their works preserved for future generations to admire? No, they are dissolved when the next tide rolls in. The artist labors over her sculpture knowing from the start that her piece is a temporary structure; in order to gain renown for sand sculpting, she must create hundreds or thousands of sculptures over many years. Build-

designed by the master | 111

ing sand sculptures is fun for the artist and for beach tourists, but laboring in vain when it comes to your life is dangerous.

Read 1 Corinthians 15:58. To what are we to give ourselves fully? Why?

_____

_____

_____

_____

Think about your progress in First Place 4 Health. Are you giving yourself fully to maintaining balance and working with God to take better care of your body, mind, heart and spirit? Or are you finding yourself repeating the same work over and over? What are you willing to do, starting right now, to produce better results?

_____

_____

_____

_____

How does knowing that what you do for the Lord is not done in vain inspire you to persevere and press on to reach your weight-loss goals, even on the days you just don't feel like it?

_____

_____

_____

_____

Read 2 Corinthians 4:6-7. If we are the jars of clay, what is the treasure we contain?

_____

_____

_____

_____

Read 2 Corinthians 4:16-18. Rewrite verses 16 and 17 in your own words.

_____

_____

_____

_____

In verse 18 we are told to fix our eyes on not what we see but on the invisible. Why?

_____

_____

_____

_____

You can be an artist laboring in vain to build something that will be washed into the sea, or you can labor over that which is eternal. What are some specific ways your focus must shift so you labor for eternal things?

_____

_____

_____

_____

> *Lord Jesus, help me trust You as together we build my life for eternity.*
> *I want to lay crowns at Your feet and spend eternity with You,*
> *knowing that what I've done here will last. Amen.*

Day 4 — LABOR OF LOVE

Show me today in Your Word, Lord, how I can serve You, worship You
and be obedient to You. Give me a fresh and passionate desire to
know You better. Amen.

Work performed voluntarily without material reward is sometimes called "a labor of love." Habitat for Humanity is a good example of people performing a labor of love. People from all walks of life give freely of their time, talents and resources to help families less fortunate than them, never expecting to be rewarded or compensated for their efforts.

Jesus Christ performed the ultimate labor of love when He went to the cross for us, taking our sin on Himself and dying in our place. As we begin our study today, let us not forget this selfless act that provided us with eternal life.

Read 1 Thessalonians 1:2-10. The apostle Paul commends the Christians in Thessalonica for three things. Let's look at each one and see why Paul was impressed. Fill in the missing words from verse 3:

We continually remember before our God and Father your _____ produced by _____, your _____ prompted by _____, and your _____ inspired by _____ in our Lord Jesus Christ.

After meeting the one true God through Jesus Christ, the Thessalonians gave up their idol worship, and their faith in God became known everywhere. Paul says that he saw their work, which was produced by faith. Do your actions (work) grow from your faith in Jesus? How?

_____

_____

_____

_____

_____

Next, Paul mentions their labor. Does your labor spring from your love for Jesus? How?

_____

_____

_____

_____

_____

Finally, Paul commends the Thessalonians' endurance. Does hope in Christ motivate you to endure? Why or why not?

What work are you accomplishing, or what suffering are you enduring, in each of the four areas of your life? How is this work a labor of love?

Spiritually

Mentally

Emotionally

Physically

*Father God, thank You for loving me so much that You
sent Your Son to die in my place. He is the hope that inspires me
and motivates me to endure when I want to quit. Amen.*

designed by the master | 115

LABORERS WITH GOD

Day 5

Father God, teach me how to endure hard times and rely on You. Help me as I learn to live a more balanced life, the way You designed me to live. Amen.

Large families, which were common when our society was mostly rural, shared responsibilities for farming, childrearing, household chores and spiritual training. Several generations lived on and worked the homestead together to bring success and harmony to their homes. Life back then was difficult and required backbreaking work, but by sharing the workload they lightened the burden for one another.

Read Ephesians 2:19-22. Christians are members of whose household?

_____

_____

_____

You are part of a large family. Think about those who are helping you along your weight-loss journey and how they help in sharing the work-load. Can you share a specific way that someone in this family of God's people has helped you deal with a particularly heavy load this week?

_____

_____

_____

Who is the chief cornerstone (v. 20)?

_____

_____

_____

In your own words, what is happening to the building (v. 21)?

_____

_____

_____

Verse 22 shows us that we are a work in progress. Think about the two phrases, "are being built" and "to become." What do they say to you concerning where you are in your journey to finding balance in all four areas of your life?

Turn to 2 Corinthians 6:1. Paul urged his fellow workers to not receive God's grace in vain. What do you think he meant by this?

Some claim to have Jesus as their Cornerstone, but their life shows little sign of building progress. When you joined First Place 4 Health, you decided to partner with God to bring your life into better balance. Do you feel that you are one of God's fellow workers? Explain what you mean.

List some of the ways you have made progress working together with God during this session of First Place 4 Health.

Thinking now about the list above, are there some areas where you could cooperate more with God? If so, put a star next to them and ask God to help you improve in these areas.

Lord, I know that building requires lifestyle changes on my part.
Help me be patient as You work on the inside and give me
endurance to keep on doing what You ask of me. Amen.

REFLECTION AND APPLICATION

Day
6

God Almighty, You hold the blueprint for my life in Your hands.
You know all the right materials and good work that will bring
it all together for eternity. Help me see Your vision for me. Amen.

Today is an exercise in vision. The Master Builder of the Universe designed your life. Think about a set of blueprints for a house. If you've never seen blueprints up close, do a search for images on the Internet or visit your local library. When you have a clear picture in your mind, create a "blueprint" in your journal of your First Place 4 Health progress, from the day you began through today and beyond, to where you finally reach your goal. Be creative as you sketch. See yourself at your goal, as God sees you. Gather some markers/clip art/stickers and whatever tools will help express:

- Who you were
- Who you are
- Who you will become

There is no wrong way to make your blueprint (except to not do one!). Don't be afraid to be creative and express yourself with color. Go outside the lines and include whatever God wants you to see. Try to show where you started working together with God and what it will be like when you are complete in Christ. You may want to include the things

God has removed from your life, the new additions He has put in and the landscaping still to come. Remember the rooms in your house and what they will be used for. Has God blessed you with things you asked Him for? If you're not sure what your design looks like, ask God to give you a glimpse. Thank Him for bringing you to where you are, and then commit to working diligently with Him as together you move closer to your completion. Feel free to share your blueprint in class at your next meeting.

Father, show me the vision You have for my life, and help me to put a glimpse of it on paper. I commit to You today and am willing to do my part. Amen.

Day 7

REFLECTION AND APPLICATION

Glorious Savior, help me continue working to reach my goals. Help me keep the vision so that I don't grow weary. Amen.

Building a house—or building anything—requires physical strength and stamina. God designed us to be balanced so that we would be able to stand up under the rigors of daily work. Perhaps you have neglected to maintain your physical body to the point that even the slightest exertion tires you, or maybe you have a disability that hinders your activity. God knows your design and He will provide a way for you to work with Him to strengthen your body. You may need to visit your doctor to determine a level of physical activity that you can do consistently, or you may just need to get up and get moving. Whatever level you are at, ask the Lord today to help you take the next step and do it!

Haggai 1:8 says, "Go up into the mountains and bring down timber and build the house, so that I may take pleasure in it and be honored." Underline the three commands in this verse. These are action verbs, meaning that an action must happen. Use each of these words to describe something you can do today or in the coming week to physically begin working with God to rebuild your temple. You can do this exercise in your journal or on the lines below.

I will go . . . TO FiRST PLACE A HEALTH CLASS

I will bring . . . MY BOOK & PEN

I will build . . . STRENGTH IN MY LEFTSIDE

Why should you take action? The rest of the verse says, "so that I [God] may take pleasure in it and be honored." How will you please and honor God today? Where will you go? Perhaps you could go on a walk with Him and admire His handiwork in the natural world. What will you bring? Could you bring a lonely friend along when you run your errands? What will you build? Maybe you could build a menu for the week ahead, and do your shopping to get prepared. Once you have decided where you will go and what you will bring and build, spend some time in prayer, asking for God's strength to help you follow through.

God, I am honored to call my body Your temple! Help me to get stronger so I can fulfill my responsibilities as a member of Your household. Amen.

Note

1. Mike Brewster, "Frank Lloyd Wright: America's Architect," Business Week, July 28, 2004. http://www.businessweek.com/bwdaily/dnflash/jul2004/nf20040728 _3153_db078.htm (accessed October 2009).

Group Prayer Requests

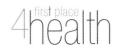

Today's Date: _____

Name	Request

Results

_____
_____
_____
_____

Week Nine

living the good life

SCRIPTURE MEMORY VERSE
Who is wise and understanding among you?
Let him show it by his good life, by deeds done
in the humility that comes from wisdom.
JAMES 3:13

There is an old nursery rhyme called "A Wise Old Owl." It goes like this:

A wise old owl lived in an oak
The more he saw the less he spoke
The less he spoke the more he heard.
Why can't we be like that wise old bird?

Since ancient times, people have seen the owl as a symbol of wisdom. With their keen, serious eyes and long life spans, it is easy to imagine that owls have seen it all. While the old owl may not in fact be wise, the nursery rhyme may offer some wisdom that will help us become a bit wiser with deeper understanding.

In this week's Scripture memory verse, James asks who considers themselves wise, and then outlines the characteristics of wisdom in a person's life; he doesn't wait for an answer to his rhetorical question. This week we will explore those characteristics so that we can answer for ourselves James's question. The picture of the "good life" James sketches here is one of depth and balance, not fun and games. He suggests earlier in his letter that we should be quick to listen, slow to speak and slow to become angry (James 1:19). The Bible, especially Proverbs, which we'll look at later, contains many verses concerning wisdom and understanding. James associates them with being evidence of our living a good life before God.

Day 1

KEEN SENSES

Jesus, give me keen eyes and ears that I might focus on seeing and hearing You through Your Word. Amen.

Many owls are active only at night. Because of their keen senses of sight and hearing, they can hunt successfully in dim light or in the dark. An owl must turn its head in order to see in any direction other than straight ahead. It can turn its head completely around so that it can see directly behind it. God gave the owl these keen abilities so that it can survive and thrive.

The word "keen" means *acute, sharp, alert* or *quick*. It can also mean that someone is eager or ardent about something. If we are to achieve our goals in First Place 4 Health, we must have keen senses to look out for things that sneak up from behind and threaten to trip us up. Staying alert to potential dangers and being eager to follow God's plan are keys to surviving and thriving. Whatever our circumstances—dim light or dark—we will live successfully if we allow God to develop our keenness according to His nature.

The question James asks in our memory verse this week concerns being wise and having understanding. Look up these two adjectives in a dictionary and write the meanings below.

Wise

_____

_____

_____

living the good life | 123

Understanding

_____
_____
_____

Being wise is more than possesing knowledge; simply having knowledge does not make a person wise. Wisdom involves balancing knowledge with good judgement. Turn to Psalm 119:65-66 and jot down in your own words what the writer wanted God to teach him.

_____
_____
_____
_____

Understanding means having a realization about something. It means that you grasp the true meaning. Proverbs has a lot to say about the importance of understanding. Find the following Scriptures in Proverbs and make a note of key things about understanding.

Proverbs 3:5

_____
_____
_____

Proverbs 4:7

_____
_____
_____

Proverbs 10:23

_____
_____
_____

124 | week nine

Proverbs 11:12

_____

_____

_____

Proverbs 15:21

_____

_____

_____

Looking back at your definitions of both *wise* and *understanding*, how can this information help you achieve better balance in your life?

_____

_____

_____

_____

Heavenly Father, I trust You to teach me how to be wise and understanding. Help me to grow in these qualities in all areas of my life. Amen.

Day 2 — THE WISE ARE PREPARED

Precious Jesus, You have much to teach me about being wise. Open my eyes that I might see, know and understand. Amen.

Every former Boy Scout knows the motto: "Be prepared." The founder of Scouting, Robert Baden-Powell, was once asked what a scout should be prepared for. "Why, for any old thing," he said. Yes, Scouts should be prepared for emergencies, but also to meet head-on any struggle or challenge that might come their way. Baden-Powell hoped that boys would grow into adults who were ready in mind, heart and body to become productive citizens and bring happiness into the lives of others. His vision was that Scouts would be prepared for life!

living the good life | 125

Being prepared is wise advice for us as well. We have learned that Satan is always prowling around looking for someone to devour; if we are wise, we will be prepared for his attacks well in advance.

Can you think of a recent occasion when you were doing great on the Live It Plan, exercising and enjoying weekly weight loss, but then something jumped in your path and you fell into temptation? Describe it, then add how you might have prepared for it in advance. How might the results have been different if you had prepared?

Look at Matthew 25:1-13 and read the Parable of the Ten Virgins. The 10 virgins went out to meet the bridegroom. Five were foolish and five were wise. What made the first five foolish (v. 3)?

What did the wise virgins do (v. 4)?

Describe in your words what happened in verses 6-12.

This month in First Place 4 Health, have you done anything foolish and felt the door to success slam shut? Be specific.

_____

_____

_____

_____

How have you made preparations to set yourself up to succeed? Circle all that apply (adding anything not included below).

Spent time with Jesus   Prayed

Planned meals in advanced   Learned to read food labels

Did my Bible study   Memorized Scripture

Asked someone for help   Went to bed earlier

Cleaned out junk and unhealthy   Other _____
    food from hidden places

Exercised consistently   _____

                                              _____

Which of the above haven't you done? Underline them and make plans to include them in your daily activity this week. Remember that being wise balances knowledge and good judgement, and that the wise are prepared for "any old thing" that may happen. Being wise is using the knowledge and good judgement that God has given you to be prepared for life.

Jesus, help me be prepared by getting my body in the best physical condition possible so that I can do the work You intend for me to do. Amen.

Day 3 — FOREST VERSUS THE TREES

Father, I want my life to demonstrate that I am wise and understanding. Help me to see the beauty of the forest instead of just one tree. Amen.

The age-old phrase "can't see the forest for the trees" has been used in a myriad of situations, from politics to finance to ecological conservation.

living the good life | 127

Political people work for their own agendas and lose sight of the good of the country. A spouse wants to win a battle only to lose the war that ravaged their marriage. Drug manufacturers pushing their product get blinded by dollar signs and ignore the welfare of their customers. Any time we are so focused on the immediate gratification of our desires, our view of the forest—the big picture—is obscured.

Scripture gives us an example of a forest-for-the-trees mentality. Read Numbers 13:17-31. God promised to give the land of Canaan to the Israelites, and instructed Moses to send a leader from each tribe to explore it. They were told to see what the land was like, bring back some of its fruit and determine if the people were strong or weak, few or many. After 40 days they returned. According to verses 26-27, what did they find?

_____

_____

_____

_____

_____

Read verses 28-31. In your own words, describe the "trees" that obscured the explorers' vision of the forest.

_____

_____

_____

_____

Have you ever felt that, even though God has promised you a Canaan (healthy body, balanced life), there are too many giants waiting to devour you? Name your giants and describe your feelings regarding them.

_____

_____

_____

_____

128 | week nine

Read Numbers 14:1-4. According to verse 4, what was the Israelites' solution to the problem?

_____

_____

_____

_____

_____

Have you ever felt that you would be better off going back to where you were? If so, why?

_____

_____

_____

_____

_____

God's way isn't always easy, but it is always right. He has a plan for you and He sees the forest of your future. If you allow yourself to focus on a clump of trees and become obsessed and fearful, you will miss all that God has waiting for you. Read Numbers 14:5-9 to find out what Joshua and Caleb, two of the explorers, told the Israelite assembly. Who will lead them and what will he do (v. 8)?

_____

_____

_____

_____

_____

What are the Israelites told *not* to do in verse 9?

_____

_____

_____

_____

living the good life | 129

Has fear or rebellion trapped you into seeing the trees instead of the forest? What action will you take today to put your trust in the Lord?

_____

_____

_____

_____

Oh Father, Your promise to me is great, but I have doubted that I would see it
fulfilled. I have focused on a clump of trees. Help me see the forest. Amen.

DEEDS BALANCED BY HUMILITY

Day 4

Lord, what deeds I do, I pray they are all done in humility
and are pleasing to You. Amen.

The term "the good life" has become a catch-all phrase for doing whatever feels good. It has been used in songs, television series, films, plays and books; it was even the original slogan for the state of Nebraska! So far this week, we have discovered what it means, according to Scripture, to be wise and full of understanding. Now let's look at God's perspective on "the good life."

Read 1 Peter 2:12. In your own words, what should be the result of living a good life?

_____

_____

_____

_____

How might your good life inspire those around you to glorify God?

_____

_____

_____

_____

Read Micah 6:8. In your own words, describe the three components of a good life, according to God.

_____

_____

_____

_____

How is seeking balance in the four areas of your life related to living "the good life"?

_____

_____

_____

_____

In Ephesians 2:8-9, we read that we are saved by grace through our faith in Christ Jesus, not by any works of our own; salvation is a gift from God. Verse 9 says that we are not saved by good works "so that no one can boast." How do you think that boasting might undermine your ability to live God's version of "the good life"?

_____

_____

_____

_____

Our Scripture memory verse reminds us that our good deeds should be done "in the humility that comes from wisdom." Do you struggle with being humble? How can knowing that you cannot earn salvation help you be more humble?

_____

_____

_____

_____

*God, I know that I am saved by grace through faith in Your Son,
Jesus Christ. I want to show my love for You by doing good deeds
and living the kind of life that exhibits Your character. Amen.*

ETERNAL LIFE Day 5

*Lord Jesus, my Savior, thank You for taking my place on the cross
and providing me a place in heaven eternally. Amen.*

"The good life" here on earth is nothing compared to the life Jesus Christ
has provided for us in heaven. He died for all who have placed our faith
in Him, but He also died for those who have not. God wants everyone to
have eternal life (see 1 Timothy 2:4-5), yet not everyone will. Many will
miss out on the glory of heaven simply because they aren't willing to
humble themselves and ask Jesus Christ into their lives.

Read 2 Timothy 3:14-15. What can the Scriptures make you wise for?

_____

_____

_____

_____

How are we made wise for salvation (v. 15)?

_____

_____

_____

_____

Read Mark 16:16 and answer the question, Who will be saved?

_____

_____

_____

_____

week nine

In First Place 4 Health, you are encouraged to read the Scriptures and study God's Word. As you continue this discipline and it becomes an integral part of your life, you will develop into the wise and understanding person that James talks about in this week's memory verse. Ezra 7:6,10 provides another clue to the benefit of studying the Scriptures. Underline or highlight the phrase from verse 6 that explains one result of studying Scripture:

> [Ezra] was a teacher well versed in the Law of Moses, which the Lord, the God of Israel, had given. The king had granted him everything he asked, for the hand of the Lord his God was on him.

Verse 10 tells us: "For Ezra had devoted himself to the study and observance of the Law of the LORD, and to teaching its decrees and laws in Israel." In your own words, how did Ezra become so knowledgeable concerning the Scriptures?

_____

_____

_____

_____

Sometimes it's tempting to think we know it all. Read Matthew 18:1-4. Jesus tells us the secret to becoming great in His kingdom. What are some ways you can "become like a little child" when it comes to studying God's Word?

_____

_____

_____

_____

_____

Oh God, give me a humble spirit to learn all I can about You
and wisdom to help others know how they too can have eternal life. Amen.

living the good life | 133

REFLECTION AND APPLICATION

Show me, Lord, what I can do today to use the wisdom and understanding I've gained this week in a way that will honor You. Amen.

Day
6

Pretend for a moment that your future is a forest, and you are on a journey to that wonderful place God designed just for you. It holds all that will satisfy your heart's desire and meet your every need. That forest is your personal Canaan, where being healthy and fit is a way of life—not just physically but mentally, emotionally and spiritually as well.

You approach the forest, but just as you are about to step onto the footpath, you notice a clump of trees blocking your way. A voice in the back of your mind whispers that you can't enter your forest because this clump of trees is in your way. Perhaps later next week, someone will cut them down and haul them away . . . *then* you will enter the forest and begin your journey to Canaan. You begin to question whether God promised the land to you after all. You turn around and head back to your safety zone, thinking about that huge clump of trees and how threatening it looked. You were so intimidated that now you need to find some comfort food to help you settle down.

Have you identified your clump of trees? You know, the ones that stop you in your tracks and cause you to question God? Take time today to name your clump of trees. What is it that you feel is blocking your path in your journey toward your forest, your Promised Land? You may have several clumps of trees preventing forward motion. Circle each one that intimidates you below, and add any not on the list.

Fear of success	Certain people	Physical disability
Fear of failure	Lack of motivation	Laziness
Low self-esteem	Unwillingness to change	Pride
Other _____	_____	_____

Once you have named your clump of trees, go to the Lord in prayer and share your fears and feelings. Be honest and ask Him to help you see those trees as part of the forest He has promised you. Ask Him to change your perspective so that you begin to see them not as obstacles but as features of your journey's landscape, planted there to challenge you and grow your character.

God, You know what holds me back and blocks my path toward the healthy life I seek. Show me how to move forward. Amen.

Day 7
REFLECTION AND APPLICATION

Lord, I come humbly before You, seeking Your face. I know that no one but You can guide me safely through the obstacles to success. Amen.

Living a good life God's way requires consistant, daily prayer. You have been given much to pray about this week, so today turn to Psalm 25 and read a wonderful prayer for guidance that you can pray in your own words.

In this beautiful psalm, David prays about his inner being, his emotional state, his spiritual condition and his attitude. He chooses to trust God instead of worrying about a clump of trees. Read through David's prayer and highlight the words "me," "my" and "I." Place yourself into the psalm. Notice David's desire to be teachable, wanting God to change him; take note of his confidence that God will act on the basis of His promises and the hope David has placed in God. Do you want to have the same attitude?

After you read through and meditate on this prayer, write a prayer in the space below or in your journal. Think about your First Place 4 Health journey and consider a week you've had recently that has been overly difficult for you. Take your time and make it your prayer to God.

You may want to begin studying other prayers in the Bible. Listed below are just a few to get you started.

1. Psalm 51—David's prayer for pardon and confession of sin
2. Nehemiah 1:1–2:9—Nehemiah's prayer for success
3. Ephesians 1:15-23; 3:14-21—Paul's prayer for the Ephesian believers
4. John 17—Prayers of Jesus for Himself, His disciples and all believers

Help me, God, to trust You in every area of my life. Help me to know the difference between living "the good life" according to the world and living a good life that truly pleases You. Thank You, Lord. Amen.

Group Prayer Requests

first place
4health

Today's Date: _____

Name	Request

Results

_____
_____
_____
_____
_____

Week Ten

your weakness, God's power

SCRIPTURE MEMORY VERSE
*Some trust in chariots and some in horses,
but we trust in the name of the LORD our God.*
PSALM 20:7

Solar energy is popular today because of electricity savings and contributions to a cleaner environment. Solar panels are placed where they can receive full sun during the day; the power they store is then released when it is needed most. Satellites store solar energy while on the sunny side of the planet, and then use that energy when on the dark side. Closer to home, solar energy is used to power a growing number of things, from outdoor Christmas lights to skyscrapers.

Think of yourself as a solar light. Left in the box or sitting in the shade, you are weak and unable to shine. But if you bask in the *Son* and absorb the power that He provides, when night falls you can use that energy and power to find your way through the darkness. Daily exposure to the Son is vital; neglecting time with Him brings weakness and an inability to find your way through the dark nights that will surely come.

We must all learn to trust God to be the Source of our power. No matter what the circumstances, it is important to stand in His presence and allow Him to fill our weakness with His power. In each area of our lives, His power will infuse us so that we are able to accomplish His purpose. Trusting anyone or anything other than God to make us strong enough to resist Satan or survive difficulty will only lead to failure.

week ten

Day 1

CHARIOTS AND HORSES

Almighty and powerful God, I come to You as a weak vessel and ask You to fill me with Your power. Amen.

The world is littered with symbols of power: monuments, idols, flags, robes, titles and, of course, money. Presidents, kings and companies compete to exert power over each other. To them, power is about dominance, conflict and possessions. They all desire to be the leader, which results in conflict that continues until one takes control—only to repeat the destructive cycle through generations.

In biblical times, the Canaanite armies took great pride in their chariots and horses. The chariots, made of iron, were virtually indestructible. Pulled by mighty horses, the Canaanites dominated other armies; their chariots and horses were symbols of power and glory throughout the ancient world.

This week we will uncover "chariots and horses" that threaten to defeat us and strip us of our power. We will look to God for His strength and supernatural power to destroy anything that threatens to carry us away from our goals. We must face our fears and trust God as He goes to battle for us.

Read Joshua 17:16-18. The people of Joseph (the Israelites) could have enjoyed living in a larger territory by going up into the forest and clearing land for themselves. But in verse 16, they expressed their fears. What were they afraid of?

_____

_____

_____

_____

Canaanite chariots pulled by horses were some of the most advanced weapons at that time. A speeding chariot pulled by charging horses left Israelite foot soliders powerless in battle. Have you encountered something that brings fear when you think about "clearing the land"? What are you afraid will happen if you step out in faith? Be specific.

What does Joshua tell the people in verse 17?

An example of God's power over chariots and horses is found in Exodus 14:5-14. According to verse 7, how many chariots, horsemen and troops did Pharoah take to pursue the Israelites?

The Israelites were terrified and cried out to the Lord. In your own words, what did Moses tell them in verses 13-14?

The Lord will fight for you; you need only to *be still*. Do that now as you write a short prayer here or in your journal, asking God to fight for you.

Oh God, there are chariots and horses threatening to destroy me,
but I know Your strength and power is able to deliver me. Amen.

Day 2 — MISPLACED TRUST

*Lord, help me to learn the importance of where I place my trust
and discern what is untrustworthy. Amen.*

"Trust" means *confidence, faith* or *a belief in someone's goodness.* The verb "to
trust" means that *we act on* our confidence, faith or belief. Placing our trust
in anything or anyone takes courage, because there is always a chance that
they will fail us. Material things break, and people make mistakes.

Think about your past attempts to lose weight and jot down a few
thoughts about who or what you trusted to help you accomplish that
goal. Include the reasons you chose to trust and what caused you to realize that doing so was a mistake.

_____

_____

_____

_____

In yesterday's study, we read examples of misplaced trust from the Old
Testament. The Egyptians and the Canaanites put their trust in horses
and chariots. The Bible tells us what happened when the Egyptians went
chasing after the Israelites at the Red Sea. They followed God's people
into what was dry ground only to have the waters come crashing over
them. God fought for the Israelites, and none of the Egyptians survived.
Exodus 14:31 says, "And when the Israelites saw the great power the
LORD displayed against the Egyptians, the people feared the LORD and
put their trust in him and in Moses his servant." Have you seen the great
power of God in your life during a recent battle? How was His power displayed and what effect did it have on you?

_____

_____

_____

_____

your weakness, God's power | 141

The Egyptians learned too late that God is the only One worthy of complete trust. Misplaced trust can be placed in many things and people, including ourselves, but only God can be trusted to do all that He promises in His Word. What will you do this week to demonstrate that your trust is in God?

_____

_____

_____

_____

_____

Today, Lord, I place my trust in You. Help me to remain
steadfast and to rely only on You. Amen.

TAKING A STAND

Day 3

Father, help me to be obedient and do what I know is right
instead of allowing fear or people to redirect my actions. Give me
courage to take a stand when necessary. Amen.

How many times have you gotten off to a great start, only to be persuaded to deviate from your plan?

Perhaps you prayed for your teenager to stand up to peer pressure and "just say no," but then you caved to a friend or coworker who wanted to have lunch at an all-you-can-eat buffet. Or perhaps a family member brought you a beautiful birthday cake the day after you began First Place 4 Health. Or maybe you planned to get out the door for a walk but then your sister called to tell you she would pick you up to help her pick out a gift for Mom.

Standing firm is not always the most popular thing to do, but when you take a stand to do what is right, you are standing against what is wrong! You and God must decide in advance where and when you will take a stand to stay on track regarding your health.

Look up the following Scriptures: Matthew 10:22; 1 Corinthians 15:58; 2 Thessalonians 2:15; 1 Peter 1:25; 5:9. Below, in your own words, summarize the common theme.

_____

_____

_____

Think about a time when you were influenced by someone and it caused you to get off of your plan for healthy eating, exercise, quiet time or other area. What happened? Were you able to get back on track?

_____

_____

_____

Replay the situation in your mind and change the outcome by mentally taking a stand. Do what you know you should have done in the first place. What was different about your actions and the result?

_____

_____

_____

_____

John 14:26 says, "But the Counselor, the Holy Spirit whom the Father will send in my name, will teach you all things and will remind you of everything I have said to you." What is Jesus saying to you today through this verse? What will the Holy Spirit teach and remind you of regarding your progress this week?

_____

_____

_____

Jesus, teach me when to take a stand so that I can remain in Your will.
Remind me daily of Your teachings so that I can stand for You. Amen.

your weakness, God's power | 143

WHERE IS YOUR TRUST?

Day **4**

Sometimes when I get discouraged, Lord Jesus, I want to turn back.
Help me overcome and give me strength. Amen.

This week we have learned about the consequences of misplaced trust, and have seen two examples from the Old Testament. It really is a "dreadful thing to fall into the hands of the living God" (Hebrews 10:31) when we have placed our trust in other things. Yet we can rejoice that God is on our side and fighting for us, not against us.

Psalm 56:3-4 says, "When I am afraid I will trust in you. In God, whose word I praise, in God I trust; I will not be afraid. What can mortal man do to me?" What did the psalmist do when he was afraid?

_____

_____

_____

_____

How can these verses help you on those days when things feel completely out of control?

_____

_____

_____

_____

Psalm 112 tells us that the man who fears the Lord and finds delight in His commands is blessed. Look at verses 7-8 and complete each phrase that describes a righteous man.

He will have ____ _____ ____ _____ _____.

His heart is _____, _____ ____ ____ _____.

His heart is _____, ____ _____ _____ ___ _____.

He will look in _____ _____ _____ _____.

144 | week ten

Read Proverbs 3:5. In your own words, what are we told to do? What are we told *not* to do?

_____

_____

_____

_____

Have you experienced a time in the past few weeks when you have leaned on your own understanding? If so, write a brief account, being sure to mention the outcome and what you learned in the process.

_____

_____

_____

_____

Where is your trust? Where have you placed your confidence that you will reach your goals?

_____

_____

_____

_____

The end of the day is a wonderful time to pray Psalm 73:25, before closing your eyes to sleep. Write this verse in your own words and then pray the words before bed.

_____

_____

_____

_____

O Lord, I can trust You in everything, with everything and through everything. There is nothing here on earth that my heart could be satisfied with other than You. Amen.

your weakness, God's power | 145

BALANCING POWER

Day 5

Father, Son and Holy Spirit, thank You for Your power that creates, saves and guides. I am in awe of how You come together as One even as each of You provides me with exactly what I need. Amen.

What a protective Creator we have. What a precious Savior saved us. What a powerful Holy Spirit guides us. Each one is worthy of our love and gratefulness for meeting all our needs and blessing us each day in unique and special ways. The power of the Father is mind-boggling: He spoke the world into being; His majestic power is infinite. Jesus Christ, the Son of God, went to the cross and took our sin upon Himself; the power in His blood, shed for each one of us, is beyond words. We have the power of the Holy Spirit within to guide us through our journey homeward bound. These three, the Holy Trinity, combine Their power, love and care to create, save and sustain us. In our triune God, we see a picture of perfect balance.

Read Psalm 68:34 and fill in the missing word that tells us what we should be doing with the power of God.

_____ the power of God, whose majesty is over Israel, whose power is in the skies.

How can you proclaim the power of God in your life, particularly as you continue seeking Him through First Place 4 Health?

_____

_____

_____

Read John 8:12 and describe in your own words the power of Jesus.

_____

_____

_____

week ten

How has Jesus brought light into your life?

Read John 14:26. Who sends the Holy Spirit? In whose name is He sent?

In what area of your life have you experienced the power of the Holy Spirit this week?

Christians have power to accomplish great things. Nothing is beyond our reach if we are acting through the power of God. God planned for us never to be left on our own, but to rely on the spiritual power He gives when we come to know Jesus Christ as our Savior. If we could manage our struggles and battles with our own power, we wouldn't need heavenly help. Think about some areas of struggle in your life right now and describe how you have or plan to put the power of the triune God to work to help you achieve more balance and move closer to your goals.

Father, thank You for being such an awesome God, for sending Your Son to provide salvation for me and for Your precious Holy Spirit who guides me as I follow You and learn Your ways. Amen.

your weakness, God's power | 147

REFLECTION AND APPLICATION

Day 6

Jesus, help me to see my weakness and Your power. I know You live inside me, empowering me to accomplish all that You have called me to do. Amen.

Look up the word "weakness" in a dictionary and write out several definitions in the space below.

_____

_____

_____

_____

Weakness is considered a negative trait in our world today, a flaw in one's character or upbringing. And, in fact, sometimes weakness can work against us when we believe Satan's lies about us. When we focus on our weaknesses instead of God's power, the enemy wins. List some of Satan's lies that you have believed in the past. In the opposite column, write down a way that God's power is stronger than your weakness. An example is given to help you get started. (You may want to look back over previous devotions to find a few Bible verses that tell the truth about God's power.)

Satan's Lie	God's Power
I can't resist eating cookies.	God won't let me be tempted more than I can bear (see 1 Corinthians 10:13).

Weaknesses in a Christian's life can be an opportunity for God to display His power. Look up the following verses. For each one, decide whether it describes weakness as negative or positive. Why do you feel that way?

Scripture	Negative	Positive	Reason
Matt. 26:41			
1 Cor. 1:25			
1 Cor. 1:27			
2 Cor. 12:9-10			
Heb. 12:11-12			

God wants to strengthen you with His power and make you strong. Submit yourself to Him today and watch as He goes to work building you up with His mighty power. Identify one area—mental, physical, spiritual or emotional—where you feel you are weak. Consider things that relate to your weight issues, but remember this is about more than weight. Weakness in other areas may contribute to your physical struggle with food. Once you have identified the area, write a prayer asking God to show Himself strong in that weakness.

Mental   Physical   Spiritual   Emotional

Lord Jesus, use my weaknesses to show Yourself strong so that You will be glorified. Help others to see Your light in me. Amen.

REFLECTION AND APPLICATION

Day
7

O God, I know that I am fearfully and wonderfully made. You have given me everything I need. I praise You and proclaim Your power. Amen.

Have you considered how very precious you are to God? No matter what size you are, what progress you've made or how far you are from your goal, God loves you! In Psalm 139:13-14, the psalmist declares that he is fearfully and wonderfully made and that God's work is wonderful. Do you believe this is true about you? Why or why not?

Turn to Psalm 8 and read it through, silently and slowly at first, and pausing wherever God touches your heart. Then go back and read it out loud with feeling. You might want to sing it to God as a form of worship. Let the words fill you with wonder for a loving God who wants you to freely love Him back.

As a way to praise God and to show your love for Him, memorize this psalm. It doesn't matter how long it takes you to memorize it. When you have the chapter hidden in your heart, you will be able to offer it up to God from your lips as an expression of your love for Him. Begin today and review it every day, adding one verse to what you have memorized the day before. You can do it, because you can do everything through Him who gives you strength (see Philippians 4:13).

Father, I am humbled by Your majesty and filled with love for You. Without You I am nothing; with You I have everything. I lift up my voice to sing Your praises. O Lord, my Lord, how majestic is Your name! Amen.

Group Prayer Requests

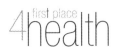

Today's Date: _____

Name	Request

Results

_____
_____
_____
_____
_____

Week Eleven

sin cancelled by love

SCRIPTURE MEMORY VERSE

*For God so loved the world that he gave his one and only Son,
that whoever believes in him shall not perish but have eternal life.*

JOHN 3:16

Have you ever written or received a love letter? When someone takes time to express his or her feelings on paper, it seems to mean so much more; we want to read it over and over. In *Sonnets from the Portuguese*, Elizabeth Barrett Browning (1806-1861) penned "How do I love thee? Let me count the ways . . ." expressing love's breadth as only a poet can do. She attempted to capture a deep, passionate and unconditional love. She wrote of loving someone to the depth and breadth and height that a person's soul could possibly reach.

God loves us that way—only much deeper, wider and higher. He loves us so much that our minds cannot fathom it. God's love will never fade or die and can never be taken from us. Romans 8:38-39 reminds us that "neither death nor life, neither angels nor demons, neither the present nor the future, nor any powers, neither height nor depth, nor anything else in all creation, will be able to separate us from the love of God that is in Christ Jesus our Lord."

The expanse of God's love for us extends through His Son, Jesus Christ, demonstrated fully when He allowed Jesus to hang upon that cross to pay for our sins forever. The gospel message of salvation is God's sonnet to the world He loves!

When Jesus paid the price for our sins, our debt was cancelled by God's love. No human can ever love you that much. If you were the only sinner in the world, Jesus would have died just for you. What kind of love is that? Eternal love!

Day 1 — NO FAVORITISM

O God, thank You for loving me. You have provided me with everything I need. I praise You and proclaim Your power. Amen.

God shows no favoritism! His love goes out to everyone equally. The Bible doesn't say that "God so loved the people with brown eyes and freckles" or that "God so loved only those at a healthy body weight." Our memory verse this week says that God loved *the world*. Period.

Read Ephesians 3:17-19. Paul prayed for the Ephesians, asking that they would have power to be able to do something. What was it (v. 18)?

_____

_____

_____

_____

How would you describe a "love that surpasses all knowledge" (v. 19)?

_____

_____

_____

_____

In your own words, what was the goal of grasping the love of Christ (v. 19)?

_____

_____

_____

_____

sin cancelled by love | 153

Read Psalm 108:4. How does David describe God's love?

_____

_____

_____

Read 1 John 4:9-10 and write how God showed His love for you.

_____

_____

_____

Regardless of where you are in your weight-loss progress, you need to understand and believe that God loves you. His love reaches above the heavens and will never fail you. He showed no favoritism; His Son, Jesus Christ, died for you. He wants you to spend eternity in heaven with Him.

Heavenly Father, thank You for not playing favorites. Forgive me for my sins and help me to show my love for You by walking in obedience. Amen.

RECEIVING GOD'S GIFT

Day 2

Father God, You love giving gifts to Your children. Thank You for the ultimate gift—Your Son, Jesus Christ. Amen.

Has someone ever given you a gift and told you to open it when you're alone? If you were busy at the time, you may have forgotten about it and neglected to open it. Can you really say that you "received" the gift? If you don't open the package, the gift is not received. When you open, discover and use it, you receive the gift.

This week's memory verse focuses on the gift God gave the world. Write your memory verse below and underline what God gave.

_____

_____

_____

154 | week eleven

How has this Bible study helped you better understand God's love and all He has done in your life?

_____

_____

_____

Have you received this gift, or have you put off opening the gift of eternal life? Read John 1:12 and fill in the blanks.

Yet to all who _____ him, to those who _____ in his _____, he gave the _____ to become _____ of God.

According to this verse, what must happen before you can claim the right to be called a child of God?

_____

_____

_____

Receiving Jesus Christ as your Savior does not mean just hearing about Him or having the plan of salvation explained to you. In order to receive Him and become His child, you must open up your heart and invite Jesus into your life. If you would like to do that now, pray the following:

Jesus, right now I am unwrapping God's gift. I receive You as my Lord and Savior. I ask You to come into my heart, forgive my sins and fill me with Your love. Thank You for saving my soul and providing me with eternal life. Amen.

If you prayed that prayer for the first time, you have received the gift and are now part of God's family. Be sure to let your First Place 4 Health leader know about your new position in Christ. If you were already a child of God, allow His fragrance to permeate your relationships and flow outward to everyone you come in contact with, so that they too will have a gift to open—a gift that will last forever.

Jesus, I'm sorry that You had to die to pay for my sin, but I'm humbled that You chose to do it willingly because You love me. Thank You, Lord. Amen.

PERISHING IS A CHOICE

Day 3

Lord, many are perishing because they choose to ignore the gift You have provided. Help me to share Your message of salvation with others. Amen.

From the very beginning, God has given His children the freedom to choose. In the Garden of Eden, Adam and Eve had access to every blessing in that wonderful and perfect place—except for one tree. God told them not to eat the fruit of the tree of knowledge of good and evil. God didn't set up an electric fence around the tree or put it where they couldn't reach it. That forbidden tree was within easy reach. God could have forced them to stay away from it, but He wanted them to obey willingly—and that meant giving them a choice.

Today we have the freedom to believe God and accept His Son as Savior—or not! It's that simple. God doesn't send people to hell; they choose to go there by rejecting Jesus Christ.

The memory verse from Week Two is, "This day I call heaven and earth as witnesses against you that I have set before you life and death, blessings and curses. Now choose life, so that you and your children may live" (Deuteronomy 30:19). What was the choice God offered?

_____

_____

_____

What did God urge His people to choose and for what reason?

_____

_____

_____

_____

156 | week eleven

Read 2 Peter 3:9 and fill in the blanks.

He is _____ with you, not wanting _____ to _____, but

_____ to come to _____.

We read in 2 Peter 3:10 that the day of the Lord will come like a thief. A thief doesn't tell you in advance when he will come, so we must be on the alert and take precautions to protect our homes and loved ones. Today is the day to choose not to perish. We need to be alert and choose to live by seeking God and asking Him to save us and our families. Through prayer, we can reach the ears of God for ourselves and our loved ones.

We can choose to treat our body as God's temple or as a trash receptacle. List some ways the body may begin to perish if not taken care of properly.

_____

_____

_____

_____

Which will you choose: life or death, blessings or curses? God urges you to choose life so that you may live longer and serve Him better.

I choose, Lord, to live and serve You as long as I have breath.
Thank You for helping me choose wisely. Amen.

Day
4

WAITING WITH POWER

My life, O Lord, is in Your loving hands. You know everything there is to know about me. Help me to be Your witness wherever I go. Amen.

Some people are under the mistaken impression that God's power is given only to overcome sin. Yet sin has already been defeated. That battle was fought and won by Jesus when He took our sin to the cross.

Read Acts 1:8. According to this verse, what is the Holy Spirit's power to be used for?

In what way has the Holy Spirit empowered you, and how can you use that power to be a witness for Him?

We sometimes get impatient and want to jump ahead of God if we fail to see immediate changes. The flip side of the coin is using His delay as an excuse for not being about His business. Have you heard or used some of the following?

- "I'm not at my goal weight, so I can't become a First Place 4 Health leader."
- "I'll never have enough money to start my own business, so I'll keep working here."
- "My weight isn't going down, so I guess I'll try that new fad diet I heard about."

Just because things aren't going as fast as we would like doesn't mean we should give up hope. While waiting patiently for God's timing, what are you doing in your sphere of influence as His witness?

What, if anything, could you be doing to be a greater influence for Christ on those around you?

Lord Jesus, sometimes I get discouraged with my progress. Help me to remember that it is Your power, not mine, that I must to rely on. Amen.

Day 5   SET FREE FROM SIN

Lord, You took my sin to the cross and set me free. Thank You for loving me so much that You would bear my sin and give me eternal life. Amen.

As our week comes to a close, let's look at the truth of this week's memory verse and get a better understanding of how it can help us. When Jesus went to the cross and took your sin debt with Him, sin was defeated and you were set free once and for all! But what were you set free from? Read Romans 6:5-18. Before Jesus paid for your sin with His death on the cross, what were you a slave to (v. 6)?

_____

_____

_____

Describe some ways being a slave to sin was visible in your life. How did you spend your money? How did you occupy your time?

_____

_____

_____

Since becoming a child of God, what are you now a slave to (v. 18)?

_____

_____

_____

How are you different? Describe the changes in your life since you were set free from sin.

_____

_____

_____

sin cancelled by love | 159

Read Romans 6:22-23. Look up the word "holiness" in a dictionary. How do you see holiness growing in your life?

_____

_____

_____

_____

Verse 23 says that "the gift of God is eternal life in Christ Jesus our Lord." Do you think eternal life begins when you die? Why or why not?

_____

_____

_____

The way to live a life in balance is to trust in God's power, not in your own. God shows Himself powerful in your life when you accept His Son and then receive guidance from the Holy Spirit. But it is up to you to choose.

Father God, because You sent Your Son to set me free, I have power to live freely right now and live forever when I die. Thank You for Your grace. Amen.

REFLECTION AND APPLICATION   Day 6

Help me, Lord, to express my love for You in my walk of obedience and in my witness to others. Amen.

The Bible is an expression of God's love for you; a love letter that pours out everything God wants you to know about Him, His nature and His character. It is an intimate and vivid sharing from God Himself to you. Think about that for a moment. How does it make you feel to know that you can read over and over again about His unending love for you? Hopefully, it will cause you to want to express your love for God in different ways.

Sit down today and think about what you have learned this week about how much God loves you. Then put pen to paper and write a sonnet to God, using the space below or your journal.

Express yourself in whatever way you are inspired; use any process you feel will tell God of your love for Him, and your thankfulness for His gift. If you are more of a visual artist, draw a picture or make a collage. Take your time and think about it before you begin. You may want to go for a walk first or spend time in a secluded place where you can feel His presence. Be sure to recount how He has helped you in the four areas of your life: mental, physical, spiritual and emotional. If you feel moved to share your sonnet with your class, please do so.

_____

_____

_____

_____

_____

_____

Gracious and loving God, not only did You provide eternal life,
but Your Holy Spirit helps me now as I walk the road to holiness
that leads to my heavenly home with You. Thank You! Amen.

Day
7

REFLECTION AND APPLICATION

Lord, my life is so different with You in it. Day after day,
the blessings I enjoy keep coming. Thank You for caring for me
by gifting me with blessings. Amen.

Don't you love opening gifts . . . especially the surprises that come when you least expect them and really need a lift? There is something wonderful about discovering what is in the package; the mystery of it all adds to the joy of unwrapping it. Many people rip the paper off and tear the box open to quickly discover the contents, while others enjoy slowly untying the ribbon, loosening the tape (to save the pretty paper) and delaying the actual opening until the last possible moment. There is no wrong way to open a gift except not to open it at all.

sin cancelled by love | 161

Your Bible is a love letter from God to you that contains many gifts of promises and spiritual truth. To discover these gifts, you need to read a portion of God's Word every day. Think of each promise you find as a daily gift.

The best gift you will find is given in Romans 6:23. Take time to look up this verse and then write it here in your own words. You may want to draw a small gift box in your Bible next to this verse as a reminder of God's love for You.

Besides the gifts you will find within the pages of your Bible, God sends other wonderful gifts to you as you walk in obedience. List a few of them here. Some gifts may include encouraging words from a friend, a phone call or the sun coming out after a storm. Gifts from God sometimes are a removal of things that can bring us harm. You may have been blessed with a gift of weight loss, or maybe you have lost your desire for foods that are harmful to your body. Habits that threatened your success may no longer be evident in your life. Ask God to remind you of gifts He has blessed you with.

Thank You, God, for the many blessings You send my way.
Every day is a blessing when I wake up to praise You and go out
to be Your instrument in Your world. Help me to remember
to give thanks to You in all things. Amen.

Group Prayer Requests

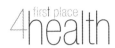

Today's Date: _____

Name	Request

Results

_____
_____
_____
_____

Week Twelve

time to
celebrate!

To help shape your brief victory celebration testimony, work through the following questions in your prayer journal:

Day One: List some of the benefits you have gained by allowing the Lord to transform your life through this 12-week First Place 4 Health session. Be sure to list benefits you have received in the physical, mental, emotional and spiritual realms of your being.

Day Two: In what ways have you most significantly changed *mentally*? Have you seen a shift in the ways you think about yourself, food, your relationships or God? How has Scripture memory been a part of these shifts?

Day Three: In what ways have you most significantly changed *emotionally*? Have you begun to identify how your feelings influence your relationship to food and exercise? What are you doing to stay aware of your emotions, both positive and negative?

Day Four: In what ways have you most significantly changed *spiritually*? How has your relationship with God deepened? How has drawing closer to Him made a difference in the other three areas of your life?

Day Five: In what ways have you most significantly changed *physically*? Have you met or exceeded your weight/measurement goals? How has your health improved the past 12 weeks?

Day Six: Was there one person in your First Place 4 Health group who was particularly encouraging to you? How did their kindness make a difference in your First Place 4 Health journey?

Day Seven: Summarize the previous six questions into a one-page testimony, or "faith story," to share at your group's victory celebration.

May our gracious Lord bless and keep you as you continue to keep Him first in all things!

Balanced Living
leader discussion guide

For in-depth information, guidance and helpful tips about leading a successful First Place 4 Health group, spend time studying the *First Place 4 Health Leader's Guide*. In it, you will find valuable answers to most of your questions as well as personal insights from many First Place 4 Health group leaders.

For the group meetings in this session, be sure to read and consider each week's discussion topics several days before the meeting—some questions and activities require supplies and/or planning to complete. Also, if you are leading a large group, plan to break into smaller groups for discussion and then come together as a large group to share your answers and responses. Make sure to appoint a capable leader for each small group so that discussions stay focused and on track (and be sure each group records their answers!).

week one: welcome to *Balanced Living*

During this first week, welcome the members to your group, provide a brief overview of the First Place 4 Health program, explain what is expected of the participants at each of the weekly meetings, and collect the Member Surveys. (See the *First Place 4 Health Leader's Guide* for a detailed outline of how to conduct the first week's meeting.)

week two: bumpy road

Most people can relate to an uncomfortable ride in a vehicle that has wheels out of balance. Ask for volunteers to describe such a ride and to be specific about how it feels both to the driver and passengers.

Ask members if any have hectic daily schedules/lifestyles. Allow time for several to share how they feel at the end of their busy day/week. On a flip chart or whiteboard, draw a wheel to represent their life. Discuss what some people may have in the center of their circle. After discussion, write

"GOD" in the center of the circle. Ask how having God in their center can provide balance during their First Place 4 Health journey.

Discuss the equipment God provides and how it will help members in their weight-loss efforts. Ask for suggestions for how God's resources will help them work with Him to become better balanced. Emphasize the importance of using these tools daily.

Ask a member to read Hebrews 10:24-25. Talk about and encourage members to share how they might "spur one another on toward love and good deeds." Ask for some reasons why this is important for your group.

If you have members in your group familiar with wheel balancing, ask if they will share how the mark on a tire is matched with the wheel weight for proper balancing (if no one knows, you can illustrate). Bring out how we should align each area of our life with Jesus as our mark.

Bring an owner's manual for an electrical device and choose a few important instructions to highlight. Have someone read Psalm 139:13-16. Discuss the passage, focusing on God being our Creator and how He knows us inside and out. Encourage members to talk to God about their weight and how to work with Him to be successful in bringing their life into balance.

Return to the wheel/tire example and discuss the value of preventive maintenance. Ask for suggestions for things members can do as preventive maintenance for their body. They may share what they wrote on Day 5 for things they cleaned out of their kitchen, schedule or mind.

Talk about protection from Satan's schemes by wearing the full armor of God, reviewing each piece of armor and how it should be used related to First Place 4 Health.

week three: balance beam

Discuss the gymnastics balance beam and focus on how athletes must prepare mentally by developing a winner's mindset. Ask for suggestions about why overweight people who have been on multiple diets have difficulty adopting a winner's mindset.

On a flip chart or whiteboard, write Paul's words in Philippians 4:13: "I can do all things through Christ who gives me strength." Emphasize that a Christian winner's mindset comes when he or she allows God to transform his or her mind.

Discuss how our lives have been changed due to labor-saving devices that result in our muscles not being used. Have members name the devices they listed on Day 2, along with one physical activity they replaced it with.

Discuss the balance beam and point out that it is the foundation on which the gymnast performs. Have a member read 2 Timothy 2:19. Discuss the meaning of foundation for a Christian.

Day 3 allows the leader to present the plan of salvation. Take time to pray in advance for any in your group who may not know Christ. Use this part of the lesson to encourage each member to consider if Jesus is their foundation, and invite any who will to accept Him as Savior during prayer time.

Have volunteers look up the encouragement Scriptures from Day 4 and read them. Remind them that God is part of their team.

Talk about the 2008 Olympics and Michael Phelps's team spirit. Remind members they are only competing against themselves, not each other, and emphasize the importance of encouragement in the group.

Discuss the five questions from Day 6 and ask volunteers to share what they wrote. (If your group is large, limit this to one member per question.)

Discuss "imperfect balance," reminding members that we are incapable of achieving perfection, but we must strive to become Christlike every day.

week four: budgeting for balance

Ask how many members in your group find it easy to stay within a financial budget. Encourage discussion of some of the challenges they face trying to accomplish this consistently. Discuss counting the cost, which Jesus talks about in Luke 14:25-35.

On a flip chart or whiteboard, make a chart with the words "MENTAL," "PHYSICAL," "SPIRITUAL" and "EMOTIONAL" written across the top. Have members call out activities or relationships that they are involved in and list them under the appropriate heading. Walk the members through the Day 1 activity of marking out, underlining, check marking and circling various activities and relationships to achieve a better balance.

Using Velcro, demonstrate how the material works by disengaging the two pieces. Point out that when they adhere to each other, they do what they are supposed to do. Ask how this illustration helps us understand the importance of working with God so the plan comes together successfully.

Discuss the risks of overspending, financially and physically. Encourage members to mention ways they can stop overspending physically (learn to say no), mentally (get sufficient sleep/rest), emotionally (limit time with negative people) and spiritually (more time with God and less "doing for" God).

Have someone read Ephesians 5:15-17. Discuss how we are unwise when we choose to ignore the Live It Plan or refuse to exercise. Then take suggestions for how we can make the most of every opportunity to properly manage our life, which belongs to God.

Take a few moments to name some perks we enjoy when we become better stewards of what God has provided.

week five: CEO secrets

Discuss some of the ups and downs of a company in today's business world, including the stock market. Ask for several descriptions of a sound company. Then ask for some descriptions of a Christian's spiritual soundness.

Go over the activity from Day 1 using the Scriptures provided and allow members to share some of their answers of when Jesus stood firm, continued in faith, showed Himself faithful, remained steadfast and knew He was secure. Ask, "Do you know that you are secure in Christ?" (Be sensitive to members who may be reluctant to answer and encourage them to speak to you later if God leads.) Discuss ways they can know they are secure.

Ask your group if any of them feel as though they have been in a rut. Pose the question, "How did you know you were in a rut?" Discuss how being in First Place 4 Health can help a person get out of that rut and begin moving forward. Ask for volunteers to share what action they took this week to prevent becoming stagnant. If no one volunteers, share something that you have done.

168 | leader discussion guide

Have a member write definitions of "credibility" on a flip chart or whiteboard as others call them out. Then compare those definitions to a Christian's life and discuss why it's important to be honest with oneself and with God in order to be successful.

Initiate a discussion concerning how dangerous it is for people to get so involved with material attainment rather than storing spiritual treasures. Make a list of material things that people strive for and then list spiritual treasures people should focus on instead. Mention the following spiritual treasures and ask how these will help them to reach their goals.

1. Memorizing God's Word
2. Prayer
3. Studying/reading Scripture
4. Sharing the gospel

Ask if members have listed additional treasures they would like to share. Discuss the reason for seeking spiritual treasures over material things.

week six: possibilities and responsibilities

Pass out an index card to each member and have them write down one thing they would choose if they could have anything in the world. Spend a few minutes allowing each member to share what they wrote.

Talk about the meaning of this week's memory verse and lead into Solomon's story from 1 Kings 11. Remind members how Solomon started strong but finished badly. Point out that he began by laying a foundation with God but lost his balance along the way and did not follow through. Ask members if they can relate to that and, if so, what is tripping them up.

Point out that having financial success is not bad, but when people forget that they need God, they get out of balance. Discuss the importance of using godly wisdom in each area of life and how doing so can help us be successful in First Place 4 Health.

Ask your group members to share examples of how the word "servant" is viewed today (slavery, mindless obedience, degrading employment, politics, and so forth). Refer back to Solomon and his motive for asking God for wisdom. Impress on members that being a servant of God is the highest order of achievement for a Christian. Talk about members' motives for wanting to lose weight or accomplish other goals.

Ask an artistic person in your group to draw, on a flip chart or whiteboard, a person with an angel on one shoulder and a devil on the other. Give an example from your own life of a time when these voices competed for your attention. Initiate a discussion of how Satan knows he can't take a Christian's soul but will try to destroy his testimony. Ask if someone would like to share a time when he or she battled between both voices and won.

Discuss the story recorded in 1 Kings 3:16-28 when two mothers brought a baby to King Solomon. Ask how he determined which the real mother was. Point out that he used the wisdom God gave him and then talk about why Israel was in awe after Solomon made his determination.

Show the class a fake and a real diamond ring (or some other example of real/fake). Explain that professionals can spot a fake because they have studied the real ones. They know the qualities of an authentic diamond and are able to pick out a fake quickly. Compare this with Christians being able to spot a false teaching because they have studied the Bible and know the truth.

Have someone read Romans 12:2 and discuss how allowing God to transform us by the renewing of our mind can enable us to make lifestyle changes. Ask members if they have ejected themselves from tempting situations recently and what they have learned in the process.

Have members consider the book of Proverbs and discuss the "do nots" from Day 7. Encourage them to read a chapter a day from Proverbs by pointing out that there are enough chapters for them to read one a day per month, much like a spiritual vitamin. Ask them to report next week on how it affected their First Place 4 Health efforts.

week seven: lawful or helpful

Begin with a short discussion on the "if it feels good, do it" attitude in today's culture. Draw members in by asking for examples. Tie this in with this week's title, suggesting that just because something is lawful doesn't mean it is helpful or beneficial to us. Be sure to emphasize the misuse of freedom.

Discuss the bondage that the Israelites were set free from and ask if any members have felt they were at one time in bondage in one or more areas of their life. Move into a discussion of freedom from that bondage, asking, "How do you know that you've been set free?" Have someone read John 8:31-36 and identify who sets us free.

Ask, "What is a stumbling block?" Explain that there may be times when we get off balance because of something someone else did; then make sure to caution that your members do not become a stumbling block for others. Provide an opportunity for members to suggest ways they might become a stumbling block in the situations listed on Day 3.

Have a volunteer read Romans 14:13-23 and then spend some time talking about prevention (v. 13). Apply this to First Place 4 Health. Impress on the group that just because God has given us freedom to do something doesn't mean we should do it when it will cause someone weaker or younger in the faith to stumble.

Have someone read Malachi 3:6 and Numbers 23:19. Ask members to describe God's character. On a whiteboard or flip chart make two headings: "God does not change" and "God does not lie." Ask for ways that members feel these two traits of God can help them know His voice and keep them from following a deceptive voice.

Open a discussion about the instinctive nature of sheep and how they listen to the voice of their shepherd and recognize him.

After reading John 10:1-5, discuss why the sheep follow the Shepherd. Ask, "How can we know for sure that we belong to the Shepherd?" Let them know that if anyone is unsure about belonging to Jesus, they can talk with you after class in private.

Ask your group if/how they can tell when a Christian is being led by the Holy Spirit and when they are not. What are some of the signs? Explore the phrase "live by" and bring out the meaning of surrender/encompass/embrace. Read Galatians 5:16-18 and ask how surrendering to or embracing the Holy Spirit will help them in their weight-loss efforts.

leader discussion guide | 171

Discuss the Day 7 activity concerning what may be permissible but not necessarily beneficial. Before closing, be sure to offer encouragement to your group regarding their efforts. Remind them that they are a work in progress and that God works from the inside out. Make sure they leave knowing that God loves them and that He wants them to reach their goals.

week eight: designed by the master

If you're able to find some photos of homes designed by Frank Lloyd Wright, display them on a poster board. Emphasize how he designed his homes to be in harmony with the needs of its owners and the location it would be built. Share that Wright brought balance into each home and made every design unique.

If you have the storybook *The Three Little Pigs*, read it to the group. Then have someone read Matthew 7:24-27 and discuss the type of foundation on which the wise and unwise man builds. Be sure to refer back to the pigs and their reaction to the wolf being at the door. Ask, "What reaction do you have when the Big Bad Wolf is at your door?" Identify Jesus as the Rock and the foundation on which to build our lives.

Discuss the sandcastle illustration from Day 3, reminding members that, even though sculptors enjoy their work and bring temporary joy to others, their labor is in vain when the tide washes in. Have someone define "labor of love" (Day 4) and ask for some examples. Offer a short prayer of thanks for Jesus' labor of love for us when He went to the cross.

Read 1 Thessalonians 1:3. Ask members to name three things for which Paul commended the Thessalonians. Have them share their answers to the questions on Day 4 about how they might be commended this past week.

On Day 6, members were asked to create a blueprint of their First Place 4 Health journey. Allow individuals who are willing to share to explain their blueprint. This exercise may be emotional for some, so be sensitive and loving. Close by having members join hands. Invite anyone who desires to pray a sentence prayer thanking the Master Builder, Jesus Christ, for the unique work He is doing in them.

172 | leader discussion guide

week nine: living the good life

Begin by exploring the difference between *wisdom* and *understanding* and encourage your group to voice how applying these qualities to their First Place 4 Health journey will bring them closer to their goals.

If you have access to Boy Scout materials, bring a handbook (if not, write the motto on a flip chart or whiteboard) and share background on the founder of scouting, Robert Baden-Powell (see Day 2). Discuss the motto "Be prepared" and brainstorm how this motto can help members stay on the Live It Plan and have a more balanced life.

Have someone read the Parable of the Ten Virgins from Matthew 25:1-13. Discuss the foolish five and then point out the success of the wise five. Allow members to share some foolish choices they've made in the past, how they learned from that experience and some wise choices they have made recently. (Always try to end your discussion on a high note.)

Explain the forest-for-the-trees mentality and ask for modern-day examples. Look at the biblical example in Numbers 13:1-33. You can also have some in the group act out the scene in which the explorers tell Moses and Aaron what they found in the land of milk and honey (vv. 26-33).

Read Numbers 14:1-4. Ask if anyone has felt like the Israelites, tempted to quit and go back. Talk about why this would not be in God's plan for them. (You may want to share Jeremiah 29:11 here.)

Bring the group's attention to the title for this week, "The Good Life," and ask someone to read 1 Peter 2:12. Spend time discussing the way God wants us to live, His version of the good life. Highlight that God wants our good deeds to demonstrate that we are wise and understanding. Our good life will glorify God, not ourselves.

Talk about boasting and the dangers involved when we take credit for what God has done in our life, especially where weight-loss is concerned. Ask members to share how God is accomplishing His will in their lives, reminding them to give credit to Him.

Ask for volunteers to share what they did for the activity on Day 6. (You might want to enlist a volunteer in advance.) Close by reading David's prayer from Psalm 25.

leader discussion guide | 173

week ten: your weakness, God's power

Use a small solar light to demonstrate how it relies on sunlight for its power to work when it's dark. Discuss different types of power and how we rely on various sources. Then look at the Canaanites and how they relied on their chariots and horses to show their strength and dominance. Ask members what the people of Joseph were fearful of in Joshua 17:16-17. Ask if any members are willing to share their fears, then have someone read Exodus 14:14. Encourage everyone to memorize this verse.

Ask a volunteer to make two headings on a flip chart or whiteboard: "WAYS" and "REASONS." Then ask members to call out different diets or methods they have used in the past to lose weight. Your volunteer will list them under "WAYS." Now go through the list and ask what attracted the member to that method or diet—what caused him or her to place trust in it? Have the volunteer write it down under "REASONS." Do they now feel their trust was misplaced? Why or why not?

Remind your group that when the Israelites saw what the Lord did at the Red Sea, they feared the Lord and placed their trust in Him (see Exodus 14:31). Ask, "Do you fear the Lord? Will you place your trust in Him?"

Spend time discussing Day 5 and assign three different people one of the Scripture passages for that day (Psalm 68:34-35, God's power; John 8:12, Jesus' power; John 14:26, the Holy Spirit's power). As each passage is read, talk about how that power can help them in their First Place 4 Health program. Remind them that God never intended for them to struggle alone.

Ask members to share how they responded to reading Psalm 8 on Day 7. If you feel led, close this time with a praise hymn to God.

week eleven: sin cancelled by love

Ask members if their parents treated them differently from their siblings when they were children. If so, how did it make them feel? Have they shown partiality to their own children? How would they feel if only those with red hair could be in this class, or if only people who weighed 125 pounds could join the church? Remind them that God shows no favoritism; He loves everyone the same. He loves overweight people exactly as much as He loves skinny ones.

In advance, prepare a small gift box decorated with a colorful bow. (You may put an inexpensive gift inside and give the box to someone to amplify the illustration.) Display it prominently. Hand the gift to someone and instruct that person not to open it yet. Talk about how we must open a gift and use what's inside to truly receive it. Have the recipient pass the gift around the group until it comes back to her, at which time she may open it. Point out that everyone held it, but only the person who opened it received the gift.

Ask, "What is the gift that God gave the world? What is the gift He gave to you?" Remind them that just hearing about Jesus or about the plan of salvation isn't receiving Jesus Christ as Savior. Have the group bow their heads while you pray, inviting anyone who might not know Jesus Christ as Savior to pray the sinner's prayer.

Talk about *perishing* and point out that people choose to spend eternity somewhere, either heaven or hell. No one sends them; heaven or hell is their choice. Not choosing heaven is choosing hell. Discuss the perishing of our earthly body through neglect and abuse. Ask members to name ways people do that. Have someone recite the memory verse from Week One (Deuteronomy 30:19) to encourage everyone to make the right choice.

Read Acts 1:8 and ask, "What is the purpose of our having the power of the Holy Spirit?" (To be Jesus' witnesses to the ends of the earth.) Initiate a discussion about how God's work in us through First Place 4 Health can help us be witnesses for God.

Ask, "Since we don't know when Christ will return, what should we be doing?" Ask for some examples of what we should do, as well as activities that could be considered a waste of time.

Compare being a slave to sin with becoming a slave to righteousness. How did members act when they were in bondage to food compared with how they act now that they depend on the Holy Spirit to guide them toward holiness?

Read Romans 6:23 and ask, "Do you think that eternal life begins when you die?" Allow time to discuss. Finally, suggest that the day a person receives the gift of eternal life is the day that life begins. We are adopted into the Father's family through His Son, and the Holy Spirit lives inside of us. Our triune God waits to receive us when we arrive in heaven one day.

Find a copy of Elizabeth Barrett Browning's "Sonnet 43" from *Sonnets from the Portuguese* (search online or check with your local library) and read it aloud. Then ask for volunteers to share their "love sonnet" to God from Day 6.

Close the session in prayer, asking God to help each member to rely on His power for everything they need to reach their goals and to live the balanced, healthy life He intends for them.

week twelve: time to celebrate!

Even though most of your meeting this week will be a victory celebration, take some time at the beginning of the meeting to talk about how much God loves each person in the group and how each of us is called to love our brothers and sisters in Christ. (See "Planning a Victory Celebration" in the *First Place 4 Health Leader's Guide* for ideas about throwing a successful celebration for your group.)

For the rest of the study time, allow each member to tell his or her *Balanced Living* story. Give members an equal opportunity to share the goals they set for themselves at the beginning of the session and talk about the challenges and good things God has done for them throughout the process. Don't allow the more talkative group members to monopolize all the time. Even the quiet members need an opportunity to share their stories and successes! Even those who have not met their goals have still been part of the journey, so allow them to share and talk about why they did not succeed.

Making a commitment to continue in First Place 4 Health is an important part of victory. Be sure to talk about your group's future plans, and make each person feel welcome to continue to journey with you.

First Place 4 Health menu plans

Each menu plan is based on approximately 1,400 to 1,500 calories per day. All recipe and menu exchanges were determined using the MasterCook software, a program that accesses a database containing more than 6,000 food items prepared using the United States Department of Agriculture (USDA) publications and information from food manufacturers. As with any nutritional program, MasterCook calculates the nutritional values of the recipes based on ingredients. Nutrition may vary due to how the food is prepared, where the food comes from, soil content, season, ripeness, processing and method of preparation. For these reasons, please use the recipes and menu plans as approximate guides. Consult a physician and/or a registered dietitian before starting a weight-loss program.

For those who need more calories, add the following to the 1,400-calorie plan:

- 1,800 calories: 2 ounce equivalent of meat, 3 ounce equivalent of bread, $1/2$ cup vegetable serving, 1 tsp. fat

- 2,000 calories: 2 ounce equivalent of meat, 4 ounce equivalent of bread, $1/2$ cup vegetable serving, 3 tsp. fat

- 2,200 calories: 2 ounce equivalent of meat, 5 ounce equivalent of bread, $1/2$ cup vegetable serving, $1/2$ cup fruit serving, 5 tsp. fat

- 2,400 calories: 2 ounce equivalent of meat, 6 ounce equivalent of bread, 1 cup vegetable serving, $1/2$ cup fruit serving, 6 tsp. fat

first place 4 health menu plans | **177**

First Week Grocery List

Produce
- [ ] apples
- [ ] bananas
- [ ] basil
- [ ] broccoli
- [ ] cabbage
- [ ] carrots
- [ ] celery
- [ ] cilantro
- [ ] cucumbers
- [ ] garlic
- [ ] Italian parsley
- [ ] lettuce
- [ ] lime juice
- [ ] mixed berries
- [ ] onion
- [ ] oranges
- [ ] parsley
- [ ] red onion
- [ ] russet potatoes
- [ ] spring mix salad
- [ ] sweet white onion
- [ ] tangerines
- [ ] tomatoes, red or yellow

Baking Products
- [ ] all-fruit strawberry preserves
- [ ] balsamic vinegar
- [ ] black pepper, ground
- [ ] Cajun seasoning
- [ ] canola oil
- [ ] chili powder
- [ ] chocolate chips, semi-sweet mini
- [ ] chocolate-flavored syrup
- [ ] coriander
- [ ] crushed red pepper
- [ ] cumin, ground

- [ ] Dijon mustard
- [ ] dried oregano
- [ ] extra virgin olive oil
- [ ] flour
- [ ] garlic powder
- [ ] jarred minced garlic
- [ ] nonstick cooking spray
- [ ] nutmeg, ground
- [ ] olive oil
- [ ] oregano, dried
- [ ] peanut butter
- [ ] pine nuts
- [ ] Ranch dressing, light
- [ ] red wine vinegar
- [ ] salsa, reduced-sodium
- [ ] salt
- [ ] Spanish rice
- [ ] spicy brown mustard
- [ ] Thousand Island dressing
- [ ] vegetable oil
- [ ] Worcestershire sauce

Breads and Cereals
- [ ] bagels, whole-wheat
- [ ] baguettes, whole-wheat or multigrain
- [ ] baked chips
- [ ] bow-tie pasta
- [ ] bread, rye
- [ ] bread, whole-wheat
- [ ] cornbread
- [ ] corn tortillas (6-inch)
- [ ] dinner rolls, whole-wheat
- [ ] dry bread crumbs
- [ ] English muffins
- [ ] flour tortillas (8-inch)
- [ ] French bread

- Kashi GO LEAN® Hearty All Natural Honey & Cinnamon Instant Hot Cereal
- oats, old-fashioned
- pasta sauce
- saltine crackers

Canned Foods
- black beans, low-sodium
- black olives
- chicken broth
- chickpeas
- chilies, mild green
- enchilada sauce
- French onion soup
- green chili peppers
- Mandarin oranges
- mushroom stems and pieces
- peach slices packed in juice
- pinto beans
- potatoes, whole salt-free
- red kidney beans
- sauerkraut
- stewed tomatoes, Mexican-style, reduced-sodium
- tomatoes
- vegetable broth
- white beans

Dairy Products
- butter, light
- cheddar cheese
- Cool Whip Lite®
- cream cheese, fat-free
- egg
- farmer cheese, lowfat
- feta cheese, reduced-fat
- milk, skim
- Monterey Jack cheese with jalapeño peppers
- Mozzarella cheese, reduced-fat
- Parmesan cheese
- Romano cheese
- sour cream, lowfat
- soymilk, vanilla
- Swiss cheese, reduced-fat, reduced-sodium

Frozen Foods
- corn, whole-kernel
- fresh green beans
- mixed vegetables
- waffles, whole-wheat

Meat and Poultry
- beef, lean ground
- ground beef chuck, extra-lean
- ham
- roast beef
- strip steak
- turkey
- turkey breast

First Week Meals and Recipes

DAY 1

Breakfast

Banana Split Breakfast Bowl

$^1/_2$ cup old-fashioned oats
dash salt
2 tbsp. light vanilla soymilk (or
   skim milk)

1 tbsp. all-fruit strawberry preserves
$^1/_2$ banana, thinly sliced
2 tbsp. Cool Whip Lite®
1 tsp. mini semi-sweet chocolate chips

In a microwave-safe bowl, combine oats and salt with $^2/_3$ cup water. Microwave for $1^1/_2$ minutes. Stir in soymilk and microwave for 1 additional minute. Stir in preserves and then top with banana, whipped topping, and chocolate chips. Serves 1.

Nutritional Information: 257 calories; 4.25g fat; 8g protein; 50.5g carbohydrate; 5.75g dietary fiber; 171mg sodium.

Lunch

Turkey Reuben Sandwiches

2 tbsp. Dijon mustard
8 slices rye bread
4 (1-oz.) slices reduced-fat, reduced-
   sodium Swiss cheese
8 oz. smoked turkey, thinly sliced

$^2/_3$ cup sauerkraut, drained and
   rinsed
$^1/_4$ cup fat-free Thousand Island
   dressing
1 tbsp. canola oil, divided

Spread $^3/_4$ teaspoon mustard over each bread slice. Place 1 cheese slice on each of 4 slices. Divide turkey evenly over cheese. Top each serving with $2^1/_2$ tablespoons sauerkraut and 1 tablespoon dressing. Top each serving with 1 bread slice, mustard sides down. Heat $1^1/_2$ teaspoons canola oil in a large nonstick skillet over medium-high heat. Add 2 sandwiches to pan; top with another heavy skillet. Cook 3 minutes on each side or until golden; remove sandwiches from pan and keep warm. Repeat procedure with remaining oil and sandwiches. Serve with 1 oz. baked chips and 1 cup mixed berries. Serves 4.

Nutritional Information: 427 calories; 11.7g fat (38% calories from fat); 23.6g protein; 57.9g carbohydrate; 6.4g dietary fiber; 44mg cholesterol; 1,029mg sodium.

Dinner

Low-Fat Vegetable Enchiladas with Salsa

$1/3$ cup vegetable broth or white wine

3 cups frozen mixed vegetables (such as pearl onions, sweet red peppers, corn)

$3/4$ cups canned diced mild green chilies

$1^1/2$ tsp. ground coriander

$3/4$ tsp. ground cumin

$1^1/2$ cups reduced-sodium Mexican-style stewed tomatoes

$1^1/2$ cups shredded lowfat farmer cheese

$3/4$ cup shredded fat-free cheddar cheese

$3/4$ tsp. ground black pepper

$1/2$ tsp. salt

8 (6-inch) corn tortillas

2 cups reduced-sodium salsa

1 cup lowfat sour cream

$1/3$ cup chopped fresh cilantro

nonstick cooking spray

Coat a microwaveable 9″ x 13″ baking dish with non-stick cooking spray. In a 10″ non-stick skillet over medium-high heat, bring the broth or wine to a boil. Add the mixed vegetables, chilies, coriander and cumin. Cook and stir for 2 minutes, or until the vegetables are soft. Remove from the heat. Add the tomatoes, farmer cheese, cheddar and pepper. Add salt to taste. Wrap the tortillas in plastic wrap; microwave on high power for 1-minute. Place 1 cup of the salsa in the baking dish. Dip each tortilla in the remaining 1 cup of salsa to coat both sides; lay the tortillas in the baking dish with edges over-lapping. Divide the filling between the tortillas and roll each up tightly. Pack into the baking dish. Cover with the remaining salsa. Preheat the broiler. Cover the baking dish with plastic wrap. Microwave on high power for 5 minutes. Remove the wrap and transfer to the broiler; broil for 2 to 3 minutes, or until the enchiladas are brown and bubbly. Top with sour cream and cilantro. Serve with $1/3$ cup Spanish rice and $1/3$ cup black beans. Serves 4.

Nutritional Information: 577 calories; 10.3g fat (31% calories from fat); 29g protein; 89.1g carbohydrate; 11g dietary fiber; 34.3mg cholesterol; 1,070mg sodium.

DAY 2

Breakfast

2 whole-wheat frozen waffles

1 tsp. light margarine

1 cup mixed berries

2 tbsp. Cool Whip Lite®

Nutritional Information: 257 calories; 9g fat (30.9% calories from fat); 5g protein; 39g carbohydrate; 5g dietary fiber; 22mg cholesterol; 577mg sodium.

Lunch

Southwestern Steak, Corn, and Black Bean Wraps

1 cup frozen whole-kernel corn, thawed
1/2 cup chopped fresh cilantro
2 tbsp. minced red onion
2 tbsp. fresh lime juice
1 tbsp. extra virgin olive oil
1/2 tsp. ground cumin
1/8 tsp. salt
1/8 tsp. freshly ground black pepper
1 (15-oz.) can black beans, rinsed and drained
2 1/4 cups chopped roast beef
6 (8-inch) fat-free flour tortillas
3/4 cup (3 oz.) shredded Monterey Jack cheese with jalapeño peppers

Combine corn, cilantro, onion, lime juice, olive oil, cumin, salt, pepper and black beans, stirring well to coat. Arrange about 1/3 cup roast beef down the center of each tortilla. Top each tortilla with about 1/3 cup corn mixture and 2 tablespoons cheese; roll up. Wrap sandwiches in aluminum foil or wax paper, and chill. Serve with 1 cup Mandarin oranges. Serves 6.

Nutritional Information: 447 calories; 10.4g fat (29% calories from fat); 23g protein; 68.8g carbohydrate; 6.6g dietary fiber; 37mg cholesterol; 818mg sodium.

Dinner

Beef and Bean Enchilada Casserole

1/2 lb. lean ground beef
1/2 cup chopped onion
1 tsp. chili powder
1/2 tsp. ground cumin
1 (15-oz.) can pinto beans, drained and rinsed
1 (4-oz.) can diced green chili peppers
2 tbsp. all-purpose flour
1 (8-oz.) carton dairy sour cream or light dairy sour cream
1/4 tsp. garlic powder
8 (6-inch) corn tortillas
1 (10-oz.) can enchilada sauce or one 10 1/2-oz. can tomato puree
1 cup shredded cheddar cheese (4 oz.)

In a large skillet cook the ground beef, onion, chili powder and cumin until onion is tender and meat is no longer pink, and then drain. Stir pinto beans and undrained chili peppers into meat mixture; set aside. In a small mixing bowl stir together sour cream, flour and garlic powder until combined; set aside. Place half of the tortillas in the bottom of a lightly greased 2-quart rectangular baking dish, cutting to fit if necessary. Top with half of the meat mixture, half of the sour cream mixture, and half of the enchilada sauce. Repeat layers. Cover dish with plastic wrap and chill in refrigerator for up to 24 hours. To serve, preheat oven to 350° F. Remove plastic wrap and cover dish with foil. Bake in preheated oven for 35 to 40 minutes or until bubbly. Uncover and sprinkle with cheese and bake 5 minutes more. Serve with 2 cups of spring mix salad with sliced tomato and 2 tablespoons light Ranch dressing. Serves 6.

Nutritional Information: 463 calories; 24g fat (42% calories from fat); 19g protein; 36g carbohydrate; 6g dietary fiber; 64mg cholesterol; 632mg sodium.

DAY 3

Breakfast
Hearty Hot Breakfast

1 pkg. Kashi GO LEAN® Hearty All Natural Honey & Cinnamon Instant Hot Cereal

$^1/_4$ cup canned peach slices packed in juice, drained
1 cup skim milk

Nutritional Information: 266 calories; 2g fat (10% calories from fat); 16g protein; 45g carbohydrate; 5.75g dietary fiber; 5mg cholesterol; 228mg sodium.

Lunch
Ham and Cheese Toasted Sandwich

$^1/_4$ cup (2 oz.) tub light cream cheese
1 tbsp. chopped fresh basil
1 tsp. Dijon mustard
$^1/_4$ tsp. freshly ground black pepper
8 (1-oz.) slices whole-wheat bread

4 oz. low-fat deli ham
8 ($^1/_4$-inch-thick) slices tomato (about 1 large)
$^1/_4$ cup (2 oz.) shredded reduced-fat sharp cheddar cheese

Preheat broiler. Combine first 4 ingredients in small bowl; stir well. Spread about 1 tablespoon cream cheese mixture over each of 4 bread slices. Top each with 1 ounce ham, 2 tomato slices, and 1 tablespoon cheddar cheese. Place sandwich halves and remaining 4 slices bread on a baking sheet. Broil 2 minutes or until cheese is melted and bread is lightly browned. Top each sandwich half with remaining bread slice. Serve immediately. Serve with 1 ounce baked chips and one apple. Serves 4.

Nutritional Information: 439 calories; 9.6g fat; (31% calories from fat); 19g protein; 71.6g carbohydrate; 10.2g dietary fiber, 25mg cholesterol; 959mg sodium.

Dinner

Greek-Style French Bread Pizza

2 medium red or yellow tomatoes, chopped, about 2 cups
1 clove garlic, minced
2 tsp. balsamic vinegar
$1/2$ tsp. dried oregano

2 oz. shredded reduced-fat mozzarella cheese
2 oz. reduced-fat feta cheese, crumbled
1 whole-wheat or multigrain baguette (8 oz.), halved lengthwise

Preheat the oven to 400° F. In a bowl, combine the tomatoes, garlic, vinegar, and oregano. In a separate bowl, combine the mozzarella and feta. Place the bread, cut side up, on a baking sheet. Top each with one-half of the tomato mixture and one-half of the cheese mixture (don't worry if a little falls off). Bake until the cheese melts and the bread is crisp, 10 to 12 minutes. Transfer to a cutting board and cut each half into 3 pieces. Serve with 2 cups spring mix salad with $1/2$ cup sliced cucumber, $1/2$ cup sliced tomato and 2 tablespoons light Ranch dressing. Serves 2.

Nutritional Information: 528 calories; 15g fat (25.7% calories from fat); 25g protein; 74g carbohydrate; 7g dietary fiber; 41mg cholesterol; 1,206mg sodium.

DAY 4

Breakfast

Starbucks to Go

Starbucks Egg White, Spinach & Feta Wrap

Grande Starbucks Non-fat Latte

Nutritional Information: 410 calories; 14g fat (30% calories from fat); 32g protein; 54g carbohydrate; 8g dietary fiber; 144mg cholesterol; 1,140mg sodium.

Lunch

Easy Three-Bean Vegetarian Chili

1 (15-oz.) can no-salt-added red kidney beans, rinsed and drained
1 (15-oz.) can small white beans, rinsed and drained
1 (15-oz.) can low-sodium black beans, rinsed and drained
1 cup chicken or vegetable broth

1 (14$1/2$-oz.) can diced tomatoes and green chile peppers, undrained
3 tbsp. chocolate-flavored syrup
1 tsp. chili powder
2 tsp. Cajun seasoning
dairy sour cream (optional)
shredded cheddar cheese (optional)

In a $3^1/_2$ or 4-quart slow cooker, combine kidney beans, white beans, black beans, undrained tomatoes and green chile peppers, beer or broth, chocolate syrup, chili powder, and Cajun seasoning. Cover and cook on low-heat setting for 6 to 8 hours or on high-heat setting for 3 to 4 hours. If desired, garnish individual servings with sour cream and cheese. Serve with one 2-inch square cornbread or 1 ounce baked tortilla chips. Serves 4.

Nutritional Information: 419 calories; 2g fat (5% calories from fat); 23g protein; 88g carbohydrate; 23g dietary fiber; 0mg cholesterol, 731mg sodium.

Dinner
Mini Meat Loaves with Green Beans

1 egg, lightly beaten
1 cup pasta sauce
$^1/_2$ cup fine dry bread crumbs
$^1/_4$ cup fresh basil leaves, coarsely chopped if large
1 lb. lean ground beef

1 cup shredded mozzarella cheese (4 oz.)
1 12-oz. pkg. fresh green beans, trimmed
1 tbsp. olive oil
crushed red pepper (optional)

Preheat oven to 450° F. Bring a medium saucepan of salted water to boiling. In large bowl combine egg, $^1/_2$ cup of the pasta sauce, bread crumbs, 2 tablespoons of the basil, and $^1/_4$ teaspoon salt. Add beef and $^1/_2$ cup of the cheese; mix well. Divide beef mixture in four equal portions. Shape each portion in a $5^1/_2$" x 2" oval. Place on 15" x 10" x 1" baking pan. Spoon on remaining pasta sauce and sprinkle with remaining cheese. Bake 15 minutes or until internal temperature registers 160° F. Cook green beans in boiling salted water for 10 minutes. Drain and toss with 1 tablespoon olive oil and red pepper. Serve with meat loaves. Sprinkle all with remaining basil leaves. Serve with one whole-wheat dinner roll. Serves 4.

Nutritional Information: 553 calories; 37g fat (59.8% calories from fat); 32g protein; 23g carbohydrate; 4g dietary fiber; 163mg cholesterol; 402mg sodium.

DAY 5

Breakfast
Peanut Butter English Muffin

$^1/_2$ English muffin, toasted
1 tbsp. peanut butter

$^1/_2$ banana
1 cup skim milk

first place 4 health menu plans | 185

Nutritional Information: 302 calories; 9g fat (27.1% calories from fat); 15g protein; 42g carbohydrate; 3g dietary fiber; 4mg cholesterol; 334mg sodium.

Lunch
Pasta Salad

1 box (16 oz.) bow-tie pasta
1 can (8 oz.) chickpeas, drained
  and rinsed
1 can (2.25 oz.) sliced black olives,
  drained
2 ribs celery, chopped
2 cucumbers, peeled, seeded, and
  cut into chunks
$^1/_2$ cup shredded carrots
$^1/_3$ cup chopped sweet onion

2 tbsp. shredded Parmesan cheese
3 tbsp. extra-virgin olive oil
$^1/_2$ cup red wine vinegar
$^1/_2$ tsp. Worcestershire sauce
$^1/_2$ tsp. spicy brown mustard
$^1/_2$ heaping tsp. jarred minced
  garlic
2 tbsp. chopped fresh Italian parsley
1 tbsp. chopped fresh basil
$^1/_4$ tsp. ground black pepper

Cook the pasta according to the package directions. Drain. Rinse under cool water for 30 seconds, then put in a large bowl. Add the remaining ingredients and mix well. Cover and refrigerate overnight (or for at least 4 hours). Mix before serving. Serve with 6 saltine crackers and 1 tangerine. Serves 7.

Nutritional Information: 451 calories; 10g fat (24% calories from fat); 12.8g protein; 76g carbohydrates; 6.4g dietary fiber; 1.2mg cholesterol; 451mg sodium.

Dinner
Italian-Style Burgers

$1^1/_2$ lbs. extra-lean ground beef chuck
5 tbsp. (1 oz.) grated Romano cheese
2 tbsp. (1 oz.) pine nuts, toasted and
  finely chopped

$^1/_2$ tsp. salt
1 tsp. dried oregano
$^3/_4$ tsp. garlic powder
$^1/_4$ tsp. ground black pepper

Place the broiler rack 2″ to 3″ from the heat source and preheat the broiler. Place the beef in a large bowl and break into pieces. Add the Romano, nuts, salt, oregano, garlic powder, and pepper. Using a fork, gently combine the beef and seasonings. Divide the meat into 4 even pieces and gently form into burgers approximately 4″ in diameter and 1″ thick. Place on a broiling pan, and cook until the top is browned, 4 to 6 minutes. Turn and cook until done and a meat thermometer registers 160° F for medium, 4 to 6 minutes. Serve on small whole-wheat bun with tomato, lettuce, and one serving of *Baked Fries*. Serves 4.

Nutritional Information: 499 calories; 26.6g fat (42% calories from fat); 38.9 protein; 27.3g carbohydrates; 2.4g dietary fiber; 95.5mg cholesterol; 597mg sodium.

Baked Fries
3 medium russet potatoes   salt and pepper to taste
2 tbsp. vegetable oil

Preheat oven to 350° F. Slice potatoes in French fry slices. Toss with vegetable oil and place in one layer on baking sheet. Bake for 10 to 15 minutes on each side, turning once.

Nutritional Information: 105 calories; 7g fat (57.8% calories from fat); 1g protein; 10g carbohydrate; 1g dietary fiber; 0mg cholesterol; 3mg sodium.

DAY 6

Breakfast
Quick Bagel Breakfast
$^1/_2$ large bagel, toasted   1 small orange
2 tbsp. fat-free cream cheese   1 cup skim milk

Nutritional Information: 335 calories; 6g fat (16.7% calories from fat); 17g protein; 53g carbohydrate; 4g dietary fiber; 20mg cholesterol; 523mg sodium.

Lunch
Turkey and Bean Soft Tacos
8 (6-inch) corn tortillas
8 oz. (2 cups) shredded cooked
  turkey breast
1 cup drained and rinsed canned
  kidney or pinto beans
$1^1/_4$ cups mild or medium-spicy salsa
  (plus additional salsa for topping)

$^1/_2$ tsp. ground cumin
$1^1/_2$ cups finely shredded cabbage
1 large carrot, shredded
$^1/_4$ cup finely chopped sweet white
  onion
$^1/_4$ cup reduced-fat Ranch
  dressing

Preheat the oven to 350° F. Stack the tortillas and wrap them in foil. Place the tortillas in the oven and heat for 10 minutes. Meanwhile, heat a large skillet coated with cooking spray over high heat. Add the turkey, beans, $1^1/_4$ cups of the salsa, and cumin and bring to a boil. Reduce the heat to low, cover, and simmer, stirring, for 10 minutes, or until heated through. In a medium bowl, combine the cabbage, carrot, onion, and Ranch dressing. Spoon about $^1/_3$ cup of the turkey filling into a tortilla. Top with $^1/_4$ cup of the cabbage mixture and fold over. Repeat with the remaining tortillas, turkey filling, and cabbage mixture. Top with the remaining salsa. Serve with 1 ounce baked tortilla chips and $^1/_4$ cup salsa. Serves 4.

Nutritional Information: 420 calories; 7.8g fat (21% calories from fat); 22.9g protein; 67.7g carbohydrate; 11.1g dietary fiber; 3mg cholesterol; 1,200mg sodium.

Dinner
Fast Food On the Go
Wendy's small chili
1 apple

Wendy's baked potato with one pat of butter

Nutritional Information: 517 calories; 6g fat (12% of calories from fat); 21g protein; 91.4g carbohydrate; 11.7g dietary fiber; 40mg cholesterol; 828mg sodium.

DAY 7

Breakfast
Crustless Broccoli and Cheese Quiche
2 tsp. olive oil
$^1/_2$ cup vertically sliced onion
1 garlic clove, minced
5 cups broccoli florets
nonstick cooking spray
$1^1/_4$ cups 1-percent lowfat milk
1 cup (4 oz.) shredded reduced-fat
   Swiss cheese
2 tbsp. chopped fresh parsley

2 tsp. Dijon mustard
$^1/_2$ tsp. salt
$^1/_4$ tsp. freshly ground black pepper
$^1/_8$ tsp. ground nutmeg
4 large egg whites, lightly beaten
2 large eggs, lightly beaten
1 tbsp. grated fresh Parmesan cheese
6 (1-oz.) slices whole-wheat bread,
   toasted

Preheat oven to 350° F. Heat oil in a large nonstick skillet over medium-high heat. Add onion and garlic; sauté $1^1/_2$ minutes. Add broccoli; sauté 1 minute. Spread broccoli mixture into a 9-inch pie plate coated with cooking spray. Combine milk and next 8 ingredients (milk through eggs) in a large bowl. Pour milk mixture over broccoli mixture; sprinkle with Parmesan. Bake at 350° F for 40 minutes or until top is golden and a knife inserted in center comes out clean; let stand 5 minutes. Serve with 1 cup mixed berries. Serves 8.

Nutritional Information: 395 calories; 6.9g fat (29% calories from fat); 17.9g protein; 61.5g carbohydrate; 5.9g dietary fiber; 81mg cholesterol; 577mg sodium.

Lunch

The Five-Minute Lunch
4 oz. whole-wheat bagel
1 tbsp. low-fat cream cheese
1 slice onion
2 leaves lettuce
1 slice tomato
1 banana
8 oz. skim milk

Spread a 4-oz. whole-wheat bagel with 1 tablespoon of lowfat cream cheese. Top with 1 slice onion, 2 leaves lettuce, and 1 slice tomato. Serve with 1 banana and 8 oz. 1-percent milk. Serves 1.

Nutritional Information: 494 calories; 7.1g fat (12% calories from fat); 24.1 protein; 103.4g carbohydrate; 14.5g dietary fiber; 19.7mg cholesterol; 684mg sodium.

Dinner

Steak 'n' Potato Soup
8 oz. strip steak, well trimmed and
   thinly sliced
1 (8-oz.) can mushroom stems and
   pieces, drained
2 (15-oz. each) cans salt-free whole
   potatoes, drained and diced
2 tbsp. light butter
2 (10 $^1/_2$-oz. each) cans condensed
   French onion soup
2$^1/_2$ cups water
$^1/_2$ tsp. black pepper

Melt the butter in a soup pot over high heat. Add the steak and mushrooms and cook for 5 to 6 minutes, or until no pink remains in the steak. Add the remaining ingredients; mix well. Bring to a boil; boil for 6 to 8 minutes, or until heated through. Serve with 2 cups spring mix salad with light dressing and a 2-inch slice French bread. Serves 8.

Nutritional Information: 387 calories; 9.9g fat (32% calories from fat); 19g protein; 37.3g carbohydrate; 6.2g dietary fiber; 44mg cholesterol; 1,242mg sodium.

first place 4 health menu plans | 189

Second Week Grocery List

Produce

- ❑ apples
- ❑ baby spinach
- ❑ basil
- ❑ blackberries
- ❑ blueberries
- ❑ butternut squash
- ❑ capers
- ❑ carrots
- ❑ celery
- ❑ cilantro
- ❑ cucumber
- ❑ garlic
- ❑ grapes
- ❑ green pepper
- ❑ jalapeño peppers
- ❑ kalamata olives
- ❑ lemon juice
- ❑ lettuce
- ❑ lime juice
- ❑ mixed berries
- ❑ onions
- ❑ oranges
- ❑ oregano
- ❑ parsley
- ❑ Portobello mushroom caps
- ❑ quinoa
- ❑ raspberries
- ❑ red bell peppers
- ❑ red onions
- ❑ red potatoes
- ❑ romaine lettuce
- ❑ sage
- ❑ spinach
- ❑ strawberries
- ❑ sweet potatoes
- ❑ tomatoes
- ❑ zucchini

Baking Products

- ❑ all-fruit spread, strawberry
- ❑ all-purpose flour
- ❑ almonds
- ❑ applesauce
- ❑ baking powder
- ❑ baking soda
- ❑ barbecue sauce
- ❑ bay leaf
- ❑ black pepper
- ❑ brown sugar
- ❑ buckwheat flour
- ❑ canola oil
- ❑ cinnamon, ground
- ❑ crushed red pepper
- ❑ cumin, ground
- ❑ extra-virgin olive oil
- ❑ flaxseed, ground
- ❑ flour, whole-wheat
- ❑ granulated sugar
- ❑ honey
- ❑ Italian dressing, light
- ❑ mayonnaise
- ❑ nonstick cooking spray
- ❑ olive oil
- ❑ oregano, dried
- ❑ quick-cooking oats
- ❑ raisins
- ❑ Ranch dressing, lowfat
- ❑ rosemary, fresh
- ❑ salt
- ❑ seasoning, dry grill
- ❑ sugar
- ❑ vanilla extract
- ❑ vegetable oil

Breads and Cereals

- ❑ angel hair pasta
- ❑ bagels

- ❑ bagels, blueberry
- ❑ bread, whole-wheat
- ❑ brown rice, microwavable
- ❑ corn tortillas (6-inch)
- ❑ flour tortillas (6-inch)
- ❑ oatmeal
- ❑ orzo
- ❑ multigrain elbow macaroni
- ❑ pita, whole-wheat
- ❑ rigatoni pasta
- ❑ saltine crackers

Canned Foods
- ❑ apricot nectar
- ❑ cannellini beans
- ❑ chicken broth, fat-free reduced-sodium
- ❑ chicken stock
- ❑ cream of mushroom soup, condensed
- ❑ diced tomatoes with chili peppers
- ❑ Mexican-style stewed tomatoes
- ❑ red chili beans
- ❑ tomatoes, no-salt-added
- ❑ tomato-basil pasta sauce
- ❑ tuna

Dairy Products
- ❑ butter, unsalted
- ❑ cheddar cheese, smoked
- ❑ cream cheese, reduced-calorie
- ❑ eggs
- ❑ Egg Beaters®
- ❑ feta cheese
- ❑ gouda cheese
- ❑ margarine, light
- ❑ Mexican-blend cheese, lowfat
- ❑ milk, fat-free
- ❑ milk, skim
- ❑ mozzarella cheese, light
- ❑ Parmesan cheese
- ❑ yogurt, light
- ❑ yogurt, lowfat vanilla

Frozen Foods
- ❑ mixed vegetables
- ❑ waffles, whole-grain

Meat and Poultry
- ❑ chicken breasts, boneless and skinless
- ❑ jumbo shrimp, deveined (1^1/$_2$ lbs.)
- ❑ roasting chicken (5 to 6 lbs.)
- ❑ turkey breast

first place 4 health menu plans | **191**

Second Week Meals and Recipes

DAY 1

Breakfast

Yogurt and Mixed Berries with Whole-Grain Waffles

2 cups vanilla low-fat yogurt
2 tbsp. honey
2 cups fresh raspberries
1 cup quartered small
   strawberries

1 cup fresh blackberries
$^1/_3$ cup sugar
2 tbsp. fresh lemon juice
4 frozen whole-grain waffles,
   toasted

Drain yogurt in a fine sieve or colander lined with cheesecloth for 10 minutes; spoon into a bowl. Add honey, stirring to combine. Combine berries, sugar, and juice; let stand 5 minutes. Place 1 waffle on each of 4 plates; top each serving with 1 cup fruit mixture, and about $^1/_3$ cup yogurt mixture. Serve immediately. Serve with one cup skim or 1-percent milk. Serves 4.

Nutritional Information: 431 calories; 5g fat (10.6% calories from fat); 17g protein; 82g carbohydrate; 8g dietary fiber; 21mg cholesterol; 464mg sodium.

Lunch

Spinach Omelet

3 tbsp. chopped onion
$1^1/_2$ cup fresh spinach leaves
$^1/_2$ cup Egg Beaters®
1 oz. feta cheese

salt and pepper to taste
nonstick cooking spray

In a nonstick skillet coated with cooking spray, sauté onions and spinach over medium heat until onions begin to soften and spinach is wilted. Distribute evenly in skillet and cover with egg substitute. When egg begins to set, loosen with spatula and turn over, trying to keep intact. Sprinkle with feta cheese, salt and pepper to taste. Serve with two slices whole-wheat bread, toasted, with 2 tsp. light margarine and 1 cup mixed berries. Serves 1

Nutritional Information: 361 calories; 13g fat (30.7% calories from fat); 21g protein; 43g carbohydrate; 9g dietary fiber; 25mg cholesterol; 911mg sodium.

Dinner

Mexican Chicken Tortilla Soup

3 cups defatted chicken broth
1/2 cup sliced onions
1 cup diced red potatoes
1/2 large green pepper, diced
2 tsp. minced garlic
2 boneless skinless chicken breast
  halves, cut into thin strips
1 tsp. chopped jalapeño peppers

1 can (14 oz.) Mexican-style
  stewed tomatoes
1/2 tsp. ground cumin
4 (6-inch) corn tortillas
1 tbsp. lime juice
1/4 cup chopped fresh
  cilantro
nonstick cooking spray

In a large soup pot over medium-high heat, bring 1/2 cup of the broth to a boil. Add the onions, potatoes, green peppers and garlic. Cook and stir for 5 minutes. Add the chicken; cook and stir for 1 minute. Add the stewed tomatoes, jalapeño peppers, cumin and remaining 21/2 cups of broth. Bring to a boil. Simmer the soup, uncovered, over medium heat for 15 minutes, or until the potatoes are soft. Meanwhile, preheat the oven to 350° F. Coat both sides of the tortillas with nonstick cooking spray; cut them into thin strips and place on a baking sheet. Bake for 15 minutes, or until crisp. Add the lime juice and cilantro to the soup; top each bowl with the tortilla strips. Serve with grilled cheese sandwiches on whole-wheat bread with sliced tomato. Serves 4.

Nutritional Information: 433 calories; 13g fat (26.8% calories from fat); 42g protein; 36g carbohydrate; 5g dietary fiber; 95mg cholesterol; 1,392mg sodium.

DAY 2

Breakfast

Quick Oatmeal and Raisins

1 cup oatmeal with dash of
  cinnamon and brown sugar
  substitute, if desired
1 tbsp. raisins

1/4 cup applesauce
1 cup skim milk

Nutritional Information: 277 calories; 3g fat (8.6% calories from fat); 15g protein; 50g carbohydrate; 5g dietary fiber; 4mg cholesterol; 505mg sodium.

first place 4 health menu plans | 193

Lunch

Healthy Minestrone

1 medium onion, chopped
1 tbsp. olive oil
2 (14-oz.) cans reduced-sodium
   chicken broth
1¹/₂ cups water
1 (15-oz.) can cannellini beans,
   rinsed and drained
1 medium zucchini, coarsely
   chopped
1 cup sliced carrots

3 cloves garlic, minced
³/₄ cup dried multigrain elbow
   macaroni
1 tbsp. snipped fresh oregano or
   1 tsp. dried oregano, crushed
8 cups packaged fresh baby spinach
   leaves
1 (14¹/₂-oz.) can no-salt-added diced
   tomatoes

In 5- to 6-quart Dutch oven (or large pot) cook onion in hot oil over medium heat until tender, stirring occasionally. Add broth, water, beans, zucchini, carrots, and garlic. Bring to boiling. Add pasta and dried oregano, if using. Return to boiling; reduce heat. Simmer, covered, 5 minutes. Simmer, uncovered, 5 to 7 minutes more or until pasta is tender, stirring occasionally. Stir in tomatoes, spinach and fresh oregano, if using. Remove from heat. Season with salt and black pepper. Sprinkle with additional fresh oregano. Serve with 6 saltine crackers. Serves 6.

Nutritional Information: 398 calories; 5g fat (22% calories from fat); 12g protein; 43g carbohydrate; 8g dietary fiber; 0mg cholesterol; 554mg sodium.

Dinner

Chicken Puttanesca with Angel Hair Pasta

8 oz. uncooked angel hair pasta
2 tsp. olive oil
4 (6-oz.) skinless, boneless chicken
   breast halves
2 cups tomato-basil pasta sauce
   (such as Muir Glen Organic)
¹/₄ cup pitted and coarsely chopped
   kalamata olives

1 tsp. capers
¹/₄ tsp. crushed red pepper
¹/₄ cup (1 oz.) pre-shredded
   Parmesan cheese
chopped fresh basil or basil sprigs
   (optional)
¹/₂ tsp. salt

Cook pasta according to package directions, omitting salt and fat. Drain and keep warm. Heat oil in a large nonstick skillet over medium-high heat. Cut chicken into 1-inch pieces. Add chicken to pan; sprinkle evenly with salt. Cook chicken 5 minutes or until lightly browned, stirring occasionally. Stir in pasta sauce, olives, capers, and pepper; bring to a simmer. Cook 5 minutes or until chicken is done, stirring frequently. Arrange 1 cup pasta on each of 4 plates; top with 1¹/₂ cups chicken mixture. Sprinkle each serving with 1 tablespoon cheese. Garnish with chopped basil or basil sprigs, if desired. Serves 4.

Nutritional Information: 530 calories; 12.4g fat (21% calories from fat); 51.8g protein; 55g carbohydrate; 2.1g dietary fiber; 104mg cholesterol; 971mg sodium.

DAY 3

Breakfast
McDonald's Breakfast on the Go
McDonald's Egg McMuffin®   6 oz. orange juice

Nutritional Information: 377 calories; 12g fat (29% calories from fat); 19g protein; 48g carbohydrate; 2g dietary fiber; 260mg cholesterol; 820mg sodium.

Lunch
Barbecue Pita
1 tbsp. barbecue sauce	1 cup chopped romaine lettuce
¹/₂ cup chopped precooked chicken	2 tbsp. diced cucumber
1 whole-wheat pita	1 tbsp. lowfat Ranch dressing

Stir together barbecue sauce and chicken. Microwave for 30 seconds or until hot. Stuff into each pita half. In a bowl, toss lettuce and cucumber with dressing. Stuff into pitas. Serve with one orange. Serves 1.

Nutritional Information: 480 calories; 11.6g fat (24% calories from fat); 27.2g protein; 69g carbohydrate; 9.8g dietary fiber; 36.8mg cholesterol; 843mg sodium.

Dinner
Quick Chicken and Dumplings
1 tbsp. butter	2 cups chopped roasted skinless,
¹/₂ cup pre-chopped onion	boneless chicken breasts

first place 4 health menu plans | 195

1 (10-oz.) box frozen mixed
  vegetables, thawed
$1^1/_2$ cups water
1 tbsp. all-purpose flour
1 (14-oz.) can fat-free, less-sodium
  chicken broth
$^1/_4$ tsp. salt

$^1/_4$ tsp. black pepper
1 bay leaf
8 (6-inch) flour tortillas, cut into
  $^1/_2$-inch strips
1 tbsp. chopped fresh
  parsley

Melt butter in a large saucepan over medium-high heat. Add onion; sauté 5 minutes or until tender. Stir in chicken and vegetables; cook 3 minutes or until thoroughly heated, stirring constantly. While chicken mixture cooks, combine water, flour and broth. Gradually stir broth mixture into chicken mixture. Stir in salt, pepper and bay leaf; bring to a boil. Reduce heat and simmer 3 minutes. Stir in tortilla strips, and cook 2 minutes or until tortilla strips soften. Remove from heat; stir in parsley. Discard bay leaf. Serve immediately. Serves 4.

Nutritional Information: 366 calories; 9.3g fat (23% calories from fat); 29.8g protein; 40.3g carbohydrate; 5.3g dietary fiber; 67mg cholesterol; 652mg sodium.

DAY 4

....

Breakfast

Blueberry Bagel Breakfast
1 blueberry bagel
$1^1/_2$ tbsp. reduced-calorie cream
  cheese

$1^1/_4$ cup fresh strawberries
1 cup skim milk

Nutritional Information: 235 calories; 3g fat (9.7% calories from fat); 14g protein; 39g carbohydrate; 2g dietary fiber; 8mg cholesterol; 404mg sodium.

....

Lunch

Chick-fil-A Chargrilled Chicken Sandwich
1 small carrot and raisin salad $^1/_2$ cup grapes

Nutritional Information: 580 calories; 15g fat (25% calories from fat); 29g protein; 72g carbohydrate; 11g dietary fiber; 55mg cholesterol; 1,460mg sodium.

Dinner

Cheese 'n' Chili Chicken

1 lb. chicken breast tenders
2¹/₂ cups drained red chili beans
8 oz. canned diced tomatoes with
chili peppers
¹/₃ cups chicken stock

1¹/₂ tbsp. your favorite dry grill
seasoning ¹/₄ cups grated smoked
cheddar or gouda
¹/₄ cups barbecue sauce

Smear the grill seasoning over the chicken tenders, and then sear them in a medium-hot nonstick skillet that you've coated with cooking spray. Cook for about 2 minutes per side. Reduce the heat to low and add the beans, tomatoes, barbecue sauce and stock. Stir well to blend. Let the mixture simmer for 10 minutes, stirring occasionally. When you're ready to serve, top it with the cheese. Serve with 6 saltine crackers. Serves 2.

Nutritional Information: 407 calories; 11.4g fat (24% calories from fat); 41.2g protein; 33.8g carbohydrate; 8.2g dietary fiber; 97mg cholesterol; 1,721mg sodium.

DAY 5

Breakfast

Blueberry Power Muffins with Streusel

To make the muffins, you will need:

1¹/₂ cups all-purpose flour, divided
1 cup whole-wheat flour
1 cup quick-cooking oats
1 cup granulated sugar
1 tbsp. baking powder
1 tsp. baking soda
¹/₄ tsp. salt

2 cups vanilla low-fat yogurt
¹/₂ cup 2-percent reduced-fat milk
3 tbsp. canola oil
2 tsp. vanilla extract
1 large egg
1¹/₂ cups fresh blueberries
nonstick cooking spray

To make the streusel, you will need:

¹/₄ cup all-purpose flour
¹/₄ cup slivered almonds, chopped

1 tbsp. brown sugar
1 tbsp. butter, melted

Preheat oven to 400° F. To prepare muffins, lightly spoon flours into dry measuring cups; level with a knife. Combine 1¹/₂ cups all-purpose flour, whole-wheat flour, oats, granulated sugar, baking powder, baking soda, and salt in a large bowl, stirring with a whisk. Make a well in center of mixture. Combine yogurt, milk, oil, vanilla, and egg, stirring with a whisk. Add yogurt mixture to flour mixture; stir just until moist. Fold in blueberries. Spoon 2 rounded tablespoons batter into each of 30 muffin cups coated with cooking spray. To prepare streusel, combine $1/4$ cup all-purpose flour, almonds, brown sugar and butter. Sprinkle evenly over batter. Bake at 400° F for 15 minutes or until muffins spring back when touched lightly in center. Cool in pans 10 minutes on a wire rack; remove from pans. Serve warm or at room temperature. Serve with 1 cup skim milk. Serves 12.

Nutritional Information: 335 calories; 6.8g fat (23% calories from fat); 14.8g protein; 54.5g carbohydrate; 2.5g dietary fiber; 23mg cholesterol; 390mg sodium.

....

Lunch
Quick Texas-style Red Beans and Rice

1 cup cooked microwaveable brown rice, such as Uncle Ben's	1 egg, fried
$1/3$ cup red beans	1 tbsp. shredded lowfat Mexican-blend cheese
1 tsp. diced cilantro	

Mix together microwaved rice and beans (rice will heat beans), top with cilantro, egg, and cheese. Serve with 2-inch slice French bread. Serves 1.

Nutritional Information: 483 calories; 10.1g fat (24% calories from fat); 17.1g protein; 58.1 carbohydrate; 8.2g dietary fiber; 214mg cholesterol; 257mg sodium.

....

Dinner
Quick Lemon Pepper Shrimp Scampi

1 cup uncooked orzo	$1^1/_2$ lbs. peeled and deveined jumbo shrimp
2 tbsp. chopped fresh parsley	
$1/2$ tsp. salt, divided	2 tbsp. fresh lemon juice
7 tsp. unsalted butter, divided	$1/4$ tsp. black pepper
2 tsp. minced garlic	

Cook orzo according to package directions, omitting salt and fat. Drain and place orzo in a medium bowl. Stir in parsley and $1/4$ teaspoon salt; cover and keep warm. While orzo cooks, melt 1 tablespoon butter in a large nonstick skillet over medium-high heat. Sprinkle shrimp with remaining $1/4$ teaspoon salt. Add half of shrimp to pan and sauté 2 minutes or until almost done.

Transfer shrimp to a plate. Melt 1 teaspoon butter in pan. Add remaining shrimp to pan and sauté 2 minutes or until almost done. Transfer to plate. Melt remaining 1 tablespoon butter in pan. Add garlic to pan; cook 30 seconds, stirring constantly. Stir in shrimp, juice and pepper; cook 1 minute or until shrimp are done. Serve with 1 cup steamed asparagus. Serves 4.

Nutritional Information: 403 calories; 10g fat (28% calories from fat); 40g protein; 34 carbohydrate; 1.7g dietary fiber; 276mg cholesterol; 549mg sodium.

DAY 6

Breakfast

Quick Bagel Breakfast

1 small (2 oz.) bagel	$^3/_4$ cup light yogurt
1 tsp. strawberry all-fruit spread	$^3/_4$ cup blackberries

Nutritional Information: 318 calories; 2g fat (4.4% calories from fat); 14g protein; 64g carbohydrate; 9g dietary fiber; 2mg cholesterol; 401mg sodium.

Lunch

Tuna Melt

2 slices whole-wheat bread	2 tsp. light mayonnaise
1 oz. canned tuna, drained	1 oz. light mozzarella cheese, shredded

Preheat broiler. In a small bowl, combine chicken and mayonnaise and set aside. Place bread onto rack in broiler pan, top with chicken mixture and cheese. Broil open-faced until cheese is melted. Serve with celery sticks with Ranch dressing and 1 apple.

Nutritional Information: 260 calories; 8g fat (27.6% calories from fat); 17g protein; 32g carbohydrate; 6g dietary fiber; 25mg cholesterol; 613mg sodium.

Dinner

Roasted Chicken with Sweet Potato Rounds and Baked Cauliflower
To make the roasted chicken, you will need the following:

1 (5 to 6-lb.) roasting chicken	2 medium red onions, quartered
1 tbsp. chopped fresh rosemary	2 whole garlic heads
8 garlic cloves, crushed	2 tsp. olive oil

Preheat oven to 450° F. Remove and discard giblets and neck from chicken. Rinse chicken under cold water; pat dry. Trim excess fat. Starting at neck cavity, loosen skin from breast and drumsticks by inserting fingers and gently pushing fingers between the skin and meat. Place rosemary and crushed garlic beneath the skin of the breast and drumsticks. Lift wing tips up and over back; tuck under chicken. Place chicken, breast side up, on a broiler pan. Cut a thin slice from the end of each onion. Remove white papery skins from garlic heads (do not peel or separate cloves). Cut tops off garlic heads, leaving root end intact. Insert meat thermometer into meaty part of thigh, making sure not to touch bone. Bake at 450° F for 30 minutes. Brush onions and garlic heads with olive oil. Arrange onions and garlic heads around chicken. Reduce oven temperature to 350° F; bake an additional 1 hour and 15 minutes or until meat thermometer registers 180° F. Cover chicken loosely with foil; let stand 10 minutes. Discard skin from chicken. Squeeze roasted heads of garlic to extract pulp; serve as a spread on French bread. Serve each with a 2-inch slice French bread, sweet potato rounds and one serving baked cauliflower. Serves 8.

Nutritional Information: 468 calories; 15.1g fat (28% calories from fat); 30.5g protein; 47mg carbohydrate; 7.9g dietary fiber; 77mg cholesterol; 152mg sodium.

To make the sweet potato rounds, you will need the following:

6 medium sweet potatoes, sliced into
 $^1/_2$-inch thick rounds

3 tsp. extra-virgin olive oil
ground black pepper

Preheat oven to 350° F. Boil a large pot of water over high heat. Add the sweet potatoes. Cook for 6 to 8 minutes, or until tender but not soft. Drain and rinse with cold water to stop further cooking. Lightly brush the potatoes with the olive oil. Sprinkle generously with the pepper (to taste). Roast for 3 to 5 minutes per side. Serves 8.

Nutritional Information: 85 calories; 1.7g fat (1% calories from fat); 1g protein; 16g carbohydrate; 2g dietary fiber; 0mg cholesterol; 22.5mg sodium.

To make the baked cauliflower, you will need the following:

1 head cauliflower, chopped
1 tsp. extra-virgin olive oil
1 tsp. dried or fresh parsley

$^1/_4$ tsp. ground black pepper
1 tbsp. grated Parmesan cheese

Preheat the oven to 450° F. Place the cauliflower in a large baking dish. Add the oil and toss to coat. Bake for 10 minutes. Stir, then bake for 10 minutes longer. Sprinkle with the parsley and pepper. Bake for 5 minutes, or until slightly browned. Sprinkle with the cheese. Mix well. Serves 4.

Nutritional Information: 52.4 calories; 1.7g fat (6% calories from fat); 3.4g protein; 7.8g carbohydrates; 3.6g dietary fiber; 1.1mg cholesterol; 62.4mg sodium.

DAY 7

Breakfast

Banana-Cinnamon Waffles

1 cup all-purpose flour	$1/4$ tsp. salt
$1/2$ cup whole-wheat flour	$1^1/2$ cups fat-free milk
$1/4$ cup buckwheat flour	3 tbsp. butter, melted
$1/4$ cup ground flaxseed	2 large eggs, lightly beaten
2 tbsp. sugar	1 large ripe banana, mashed
$1^1/2$ tsp. baking powder	nonstick cooking spray
$1/2$ tsp. ground cinnamon	

Lightly spoon flours into dry measuring cups; level with a knife. Combine flours, flaxseed, sugar, baking powder, cinnamon and salt in a medium bowl, stirring with a whisk. Combine milk, butter and eggs, stirring with a whisk; add milk mixture to flour mixture, stirring until blended. Fold in mashed banana. Preheat a waffle iron and coat with cooking spray. Spoon about $1/4$ cup batter per 4-inch waffle onto the hot waffle iron, spreading batter to edges. Cook 3 to 4 minutes or until steaming stops; repeat procedure with remaining batter. Serve with 1 cup skim milk. Serves 8 (serving size: 2 waffles).

Nutritional Information: 301 calories; 7.4g fat (31% calories from fat); 15.3g protein; 43.1g carbohydrate; 3.4g dietary fiber; 69mg cholesterol; 364mg sodium.

Lunch

Squash-Quinoa Soup

12 oz. skinless, boneless chicken breast halves, cut into 1-inch pieces	$1/3$ cup finely chopped shallot or onion
2 tsp. olive or canola oil	1 (5.5-oz.) can apricot nectar

2 (14-oz.) cans reduced-sodium chicken broth	$^3/_4$ cup quinoa, rinsed and drained
	1 tsp. ground cumin
1 lb. butternut squash, peeled, halved, seeded, cut into 1-inch cubes	2 small zucchini, halved lengthwise and cut into 1-inch pieces

In a saucepan, cook chicken and shallot in hot oil over medium heat 2 to 3 minutes or until shallots are tender, stirring occasionally. Add broth, apricot nectar, squash, quinoa, and cumin. Bring to boiling; reduce heat. Simmer, covered, 5 minutes and add zucchini. Cover and cook 10 minutes more or until squash and quinoa are tender. Season to taste with salt and ground black pepper. Serve with $^1/_2$ sliced turkey breast sandwich on whole-wheat bread with lettuce and tomato and 1 tablespoon light mayonnaise. Serves 6.

Nutritional Information: 352 calories; 6g fat (17% calories from fat); 34g protein; 44g carbohydrate; 5g dietary fiber; 65mg cholesterol; 674mg sodium.

Dinner

Portobello Pasta Bake

8 oz. small rigatoni pasta	2 red bell peppers, cut into strips
2 tbsp. olive or vegetable oil	2 cans (10 oz. each) condensed cream
1 lb. boneless, skinless chicken breasts, cut into 1-inch pieces	of mushroom soup
	2 cups chicken broth
2 large Portobello mushroom caps, sliced	2 tbsp. fresh chopped sage
	$^1/_3$ cup ($1^1/_2$ oz.) grated Parmesan
1 onion, halved and sliced	cheese

Preheat the oven to 375° F. Coat a 13″ x 9″ baking dish with cooking spray. Prepare the pasta according to package directions. Meanwhile, heat 1 tablespoon of the oil in a large skillet over medium-high heat. Add the chicken and cook, turning once, for 8 minutes, or until golden. Remove to a plate and keep warm. Heat the remaining 1 tablespoon oil in the same skillet. Add the mushrooms, onion, and peppers and cook, stirring occasionally, for 8 minutes, or until soft. In a large bowl combine the chicken, pasta, mushroom mixture, soup, broth, and sage. Spoon into the prepared baking dish. Sprinkle with the cheese. Cover loosely with foil and bake for 20 minutes. Remove the foil and bake for 10 minutes longer, or until hot and bubbly. Serve with sliced cucumber and tomato salad with light Italian dressing. Serves 6.

Nutritional Information: 389 calories; 13.7g fat (31% calories from fat); 27.3g protein; 39.7 carbohydrate; 2.9g dietary fiber; 47.8mg cholesterol; 1,042mg sodium.

SNACKS
(**Note:** Add the ingredients for each of these items to the grocery lists.)

Peanut Butter and Jelly Muffin
1/2 banana

2 tsp. peanut butter

English muffin, whole-wheat

Mash banana into peanut butter and spread onto the muffin.

Nutritional Information: 252 calories; 7g fat (23.5% calories from fat); 8g protein; 42g carbohydrate; 4g dietary fiber; 0mg cholesterol; 315mg sodium.

Bagel with Cheese
1 tbsp. part-skim ricotta cheese

1/2 small cinnamon-rasin bagel

dash of cinnamon

apple

Spread ricotta cheese over bagel. Sprinkle with cinnamon, if desired, and top with a thinly sliced apple.

Nutritional Information: 130 calories; 3g fat (18.1% calories from fat); 5g protein; 22g carbohydrate; 2g dietary fiber; 8mg cholesterol; 128mg sodium.

Spicy Roasted Chickpeas
2 cups canned chick-peas, rinsed
and drained

1 1/2 tsp. extra-virgin olive oil

1/2 tsp. ground cumin

1/2 tsp. ground coriander

1/4 tsp. ground red pepper

1/4 tsp. ground black pepper

Preheat the oven to 400° F. Coat a baking sheet with non-stick spray and set aside. In a small bowl, toss the chickpeas with the oil, cumin, coriander, red pepper and black pepper. Place the chickpeas in a single layer on the prepared baking sheet. Bake for 30 to 40 minutes, or until crisp and golden. Serves 6 (1/3-cup servings).

Nutritional Information: 80 calories; 1.6g fat; 3g protein; 13.7g carbohydrate; 2.7g dietary fiber; 0mg cholesterol; 179mg sodium.

Cucumber Salad
1 cucumber, halved lengthwise

1/2 sweet onion, coarsely chopped
(about 2/3 cup)

1/2 cup water

1/2 cup apple cider vinegar

1 tsp. Splenda® or sugar

1 tsp. ground black pepper

1/2 tsp. salt

Cut the cucumber halves into thin slices. Place in a large bowl. Add the onion, water, vinegar, Splenda or sugar, pepper, and salt. Stir to mix well. Cover and refrigerate for at least 1 hour, or up to overnight. Serves 16.

Nutritional Information: 9 calories; 0g fat (0% calories from fat); 0.2g protein; 2.2g carbohydrate; 0.2g dietary fiber; 0mg cholesterol; 73.9mg sodium.

OTHER GREAT SNACK IDEAS

(**Note:** Add the ingredients for each of these items to the grocery lists. Each of these snack ideas are under 200 calories.)

- 4 cups light butter popcorn
- 100-percent frozen fruit bar
- 1 cup of your favorite low-sugar cereal
- 30 small pretzel sticks
- Snack Plate: 25 red grapes, 3 tablespoons feta cheese, 6 crackers

DESSERTS

(**Note:** Add the ingredients for each of these items to the grocery lists.)

Pumpkin Spice Cake

1 can pumpkin
1 box spice cake mix

$^1/_4$ cup chopped walnuts

Blend and bake according to cake mix package directions.

Nutritional Information: 109 calories; 4g fat (28.8% calories from fat); 2g protein; 18g carbohydrate; trace dietary fiber; 0mg cholesterol; 149mg sodium.

Chocolate Cherry Swirl Cake

1 pkg. (18$^1/_4$ oz.) chocolate
  cake mix
1 (20 oz.) can reduced sugar cherry
  pie filling
5 egg whites

1 tsp. vanilla
8 oz. reduced-fat cream cheese
$^1/_3$ cup Splenda®
$^1/_2$ tsp. vanilla
2 egg whites

In a large bowl combine the cake mix, pie filling, egg whites and vanilla just until moistened. Spread into a 13″ x 9″ x 2″ baking dish coated with cooking spray; set aside. In a small mixing bowl, beat the cream cheese, Splenda® and vanilla. Add the egg whites; beat on low speed just until combined.

Spread over batter; cut through batter with a knife to swirl. Bake at 350° F for 35-40 minutes or until a toothpick inserted near the center comes out clean and topping is set. Cool. Store in the refrigerator. Serve with cool whip.

Nutritional Information: 207 calories; 5g fat (22% calories from fat); 5g protein; 35g carbohydrate; 1g dietary fiber; 5mg cholesterol; 350mg sodium.

Refreshing Lime Pie

1 envelope unflavored gelatin
$1/2$ cup cold water
1 package sugar-free lime gelatin
$1/2$ cup boiling water
3 tbsp. lime juice

3 cartons (6-8 oz. each) fat-free reduced-sugar key lime yogurt
$1^1/2$ cups reduced-fat whipped topping
1 shortbread or graham cracker crust

In a bowl, sprinkle unflavored gelatin over cold water; let stand for 3 minutes. In another bowl, dissolve lime gelatin in boiling water; stir in unflavored gelatin until dissolved. Refrigerate for 10 minutes. Stir in yogurt and lime juice. Chill until partially set. Fold in whipped topping. Pour into piecrust. Chill until firm. May top with more whipped topping if desired. Serves 8.

Nutritional Information: 172 calories; 6g fat (31% calories from fat); 6g protein; 24g carbohydrate; 0g dietary fiber; 1mg cholesterol; 183mg sodium.

Black Bottom Banana Pie

1 cup cold skim milk
1 (4 serving size) chocolate flavored sugar-free instant pudding
1 banana
2 cups cold skim milk

1 (4 serving size) vanilla sugar-free instant pudding
4 oz. Cool Whip Lite®, thawed
1 reduced-fat graham cracker crust

Pour 1 cup milk into medium bowl; add chocolate pudding mix. Beat with an electric mixer for one minute (mixture will be very thick). Spread mixture carefully into piecrust. Top with sliced banana. Mix 2 cups milk with vanilla pudding mix. Spread over chocolate/banana layer. Cover and chill at least three hours before serving. Top with Cool Whip Lite®. Serves 8.

Nutritional Information: 201 calories; 6g fat (25.7% calories from fat); 4g protein; 31g carbohydrate; 1g dietary fiber; 2mg cholesterol; 273mg sodium.

Member Survey

Please answer the following questions to help your leader plan your First Place 4 Health meetings so that your needs might be met in this session. Give this form to your leader at the first group meeting.

Name _____ Birth date _____

Please list those who live in your household.

Name	Relationship	Age

What church do you attend? _____

Are you interested in receiving more information about our church?

　　　Yes　　　No

Occupation _____

What talent or area of expertise would you be willing to share with our class?

_____

Why did you join First Place 4 Health?

_____

With notice, would you be willing to lead a Bible study discussion one week?

　　　Yes　　　No

Are you comfortable praying out loud? _____

If the assistant leader were absent, would you be willing to assist in weighing in members and possibly evaluating the Live It Trackers?

　　　Yes　　　No

Any other comments:

_____

_____

Personal Weight and Measurement Record

Week	Weight	+ or -	Goal this Session	Pounds to goal
1				
2				
3				
4				
5				
6				
7				
8				
9				
10				
11				
12				

Beginning Measurements

Waist _____ Hips _____ Thighs _____ Chest _____

Ending Measurements

Waist _____ Hips _____ Thighs _____ Chest _____

First Place 4 Health
Prayer Partner

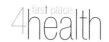

BALANCED LIVING
Week 1

SCRIPTURE VERSE TO MEMORIZE FOR WEEK TWO:
This day I call heaven and earth as witnesses against you that I have set before you life and death, blessings and curses. Now choose life, so that you and your children may live.
DEUTERONOMY 30:19

Date: _____

Name: _____

Home Phone: (_____) _____

Work Phone: _____

Email: _____

Personal Prayer Concerns:

_____
_____
_____
_____
_____
_____
_____

This form is for prayer requests that are personal to you and your journey in First Place 4 Health. Please complete this form and have it ready to turn in when you arrive at your group meeting.

First Place 4 Health
Prayer Partner

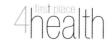

BALANCED LIVING Week 2

SCRIPTURE VERSE TO MEMORIZE FOR WEEK THREE:

Jesus grew in wisdom and stature, and in favor with God and men.

LUKE 2:52

Date: _____

Name: _____

Home Phone: (___) _____

Work Phone: (___) _____

Email: _____

Personal Prayer Concerns:

_____
_____
_____
_____
_____
_____
_____

This form is for prayer requests that are personal to you and your journey in First Place 4 Health. Please complete this form and have it ready to turn in when you arrive at your group meeting.

First Place 4 Health
Prayer Partner

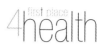

BALANCED LIVING
Week 3

Scripture Verse to Memorize for Week Four:

Be strong and very courageous. Be careful to obey all the law my servant Moses gave you; do not turn from it to the right or to the left, that you may be successful wherever you go.

Joshua 1:7

Date: _____

Name: _____

Home Phone: (___) _____

Work Phone: (___) _____

Email: _____

Personal Prayer Concerns:

_____
_____
_____
_____
_____
_____
_____

This form is for prayer requests that are personal to you and your journey in First Place 4 Health. Please complete this form and have it ready to turn in when you arrive at your group meeting.

*First Place 4 Health
Prayer Partner*

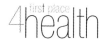

BALANCED LIVING Week 4

Scripture Verse to Memorize for Week Five:

Therefore, prepare your minds for action; be self-controlled; set your hope fully on the grace to be given you when Jesus Christ is revealed.

1 Peter 1:13

Date: _____

Name: _____

Home Phone: _____

Work Phone: _____

Email: _____

Personal Prayer Concerns:

_____
_____
_____
_____
_____
_____

First Place 4 Health
Prayer Partner

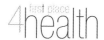

BALANCED LIVING
Week 5

Scripture Verse to Memorize for Week Six:

So give your servant a discerning heart to govern your people and to distinguish between right and wrong.

1 Kings 3:9

Date: _____

Name: _____

Home Phone: _____

Work Phone: _____

Email: _____

Personal Prayer Concerns:

_____
_____
_____
_____
_____
_____

First Place 4 Health
Prayer Partner

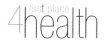

BALANCED LIVING Week 6

SCRIPTURE VERSE TO MEMORIZE FOR WEEK SEVEN:
"Everything is permissible for me"—but not everything is beneficial.
"Everything is permissible for me"—but I will not be mastered by anything.
1 CORINTHIANS 6:12

Date: _____

Name: _____

Home Phone: _____

Work Phone: _____

Email: _____

Personal Prayer Concerns:

_____
_____
_____
_____
_____
_____
_____

This form is for prayer requests that are personal to you and your journey in First Place 4 Health. Please complete this form and have it ready to turn in when you arrive at your group meeting.

First Place 4 Health
Prayer Partner

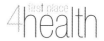

BALANCED LIVING
Week 7

SCRIPTURE VERSE TO MEMORIZE FOR WEEK EIGHT:
Unless the LORD builds the house, its builders labor in vain.
PSALM 127:1

Date: _____

Name: _____

Home Phone: _____

Work Phone: _____

Email: _____

Personal Prayer Concerns:

_____
_____
_____
_____
_____
_____
_____

This form is for prayer requests that are personal to you and your journey in First Place 4 Health. Please complete this form and have it ready to turn in when you arrive at your group meeting.

First Place 4 Health
Prayer Partner

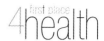

BALANCED LIVING Week 8

SCRIPTURE VERSE TO MEMORIZE FOR WEEK NINE:
Who is wise and understanding among you? Let him show it by his good life, by deeds done in the humility that comes from wisdom.
JAMES 3:13

Date: _____

Name: _____

Home Phone: (_____) _____

Work Phone: (_____) _____

Email: _____

Personal Prayer Concerns:

_____
_____
_____
_____
_____
_____
_____

This form is for prayer requests that are personal to you and your journey in First Place 4 Health. Please complete this form and have it ready to turn in when you arrive at your group meeting.

First Place 4 Health
Prayer Partner

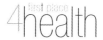

BALANCED LIVING
Week **9**

SCRIPTURE VERSE TO MEMORIZE FOR WEEK TEN:

*Some trust in chariots and some in horses,
but we trust in the name of the LORD our God.*

PSALM 20:7

Date: _____

Name: _____

Home Phone: _____

Work Phone: _____

Email: _____

Personal Prayer Concerns:

_____
_____
_____
_____
_____
_____
_____

This form is for prayer requests that are personal to you and your journey in First Place 4 Health. Please complete this form and have it ready to turn in when you arrive at your group meeting.

First Place 4 Health
Prayer Partner

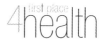

BALANCED LIVING
Week 10

SCRIPTURE VERSE TO MEMORIZE FOR WEEK ELEVEN:
For God so loved the world that he gave his one and only Son, that whoever believes in him shall not perish but have eternal life.
JOHN 3:16

Date: _____

Name: _____

Home Phone: (_____) _____

Work Phone: (_____) _____

Email: _____

Personal Prayer Concerns:

_____
_____
_____
_____
_____
_____
_____
_____

This form is for prayer requests that are personal to you and your journey in First Place 4 Health. Please complete this form and have it ready to turn in when you arrive at your group meeting.

First Place 4 Health
Prayer Partner

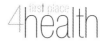

BALANCED LIVING
Week
11

Date: _____

Name: _____

Home Phone: (___) _____

Work Phone: (___) _____

Email: _____

Personal Prayer Concerns:

_____
_____
_____
_____
_____
_____
_____

This form is for prayer requests that are personal to you and your journey in First Place 4 Health. Please complete this form and have it ready to turn in when you arrive at your group meeting.

Live It Tracker

Name: _____ Loss/gain: _____ lbs.

Date: _____ Week #: _____ Calorie Range: _____ My food goal for next week: _____

Activity Level: None, < 30 min/day, 30-60 min/day, 60+ min/day My activity goal for next week: _____

Group	Daily Calories							
	1300-1400	1500-1600	1700-1800	1900-2000	2100-2200	2300-2400	2500-2600	2700-2800
Fruits	1.5-2 c.	1.5-2 c.	1.5-2 c.	2-2.5 c.	2-2.5 c.	2.5-3.5 c.	3.5-4.5 c.	3.5-4.5 c.
Vegetables	1.5-2 c.	2-2.5 c.	2.5-3 c.	2.5-3 c.	3-3.5 c.	3.5-4.5 c.	4.5-5 c.	4.5-5 c.
Grains	5 oz-eq.	5-6 oz-eq.	6-7 oz-eq.	6-7 oz-eq.	7-8 oz-eq.	8-9 oz-eq.	9-10 oz-eq.	10-11 oz-eq.
Meat & Beans	4 oz-eq.	5 oz-eq.	5-5.5 oz-eq.	5.5-6.5 oz-eq.	6.5-7 oz-eq.	7-7.5 oz-eq.	7-7.5 oz-eq.	7.5-8 oz-eq.
Milk	2-3 c.	3 c.	3 c.	3 c.	3 c.	3 c.	3 c.	3 c.
Healthy Oils	4 tsp.	5 tsp.	5 tsp.	6 tsp.	6 tsp.	7 tsp.	8 tsp.	8 tsp.

Day/Date: _____

Breakfast: _____ Lunch: _____

Dinner: _____ Snack: _____

Group	Fruits	Vegetables	Grains	Meat & Beans	Milk	Oils
Goal Amount						
Estimate Your Total						
Increase ⇧ or Decrease? ⇩						

Physical Activity: _____ Spiritual Activity: _____

Steps/Miles/Minutes: _____

Day/Date: _____

Breakfast: _____ Lunch: _____

Dinner: _____ Snack: _____

Group	Fruits	Vegetables	Grains	Meat & Beans	Milk	Oils
Goal Amount						
Estimate Your Total						
Increase ⇧ or Decrease? ⇩						

Physical Activity: _____ Spiritual Activity: _____

Steps/Miles/Minutes: _____

Day/Date: _____

Breakfast: _____ Lunch: _____

Dinner: _____ Snack: _____

Group	Fruits	Vegetables	Grains	Meat & Beans	Milk	Oils
Goal Amount						
Estimate Your Total						
Increase ⇧ or Decrease? ⇩						

Physical Activity: _____ Spiritual Activity: _____

Steps/Miles/Minutes: _____

Copyright 2009 First Place 4 Health. Do not duplicate without permission from First Place 4 Health.

Day/Date:

Breakfast: _____ Lunch: _____

Dinner: _____ Snack: _____

Group	Fruits	Vegetables	Grains	Meat & Beans	Milk	Oils
Goal Amount						
Estimate Your Total						
Increase ⇧ or Decrease? ⇩						

Physical Activity: _____ Spiritual Activity: _____

Steps/Miles/Minutes: _____ _____

Day/Date:

Breakfast: _____ Lunch: _____

Dinner: _____ Snack: _____

Group	Fruits	Vegetables	Grains	Meat & Beans	Milk	Oils
Goal Amount						
Estimate Your Total						
Increase ⇧ or Decrease? ⇩						

Physical Activity: _____ Spiritual Activity: _____

Steps/Miles/Minutes: _____ _____

Day/Date:

Breakfast: _____ Lunch: _____

Dinner: _____ Snack: _____

Group	Fruits	Vegetables	Grains	Meat & Beans	Milk	Oils
Goal Amount						
Estimate Your Total						
Increase ⇧ or Decrease? ⇩						

Physical Activity: _____ Spiritual Activity: _____

Steps/Miles/Minutes: _____ _____

Day/Date:

Breakfast: _____ Lunch: _____

Dinner: _____ Snack: _____

Group	Fruits	Vegetables	Grains	Meat & Beans	Milk	Oils
Goal Amount						
Estimate Your Total						
Increase ⇧ or Decrease? ⇩						

Physical Activity: _____ Spiritual Activity: _____

Steps/Miles/Minutes: _____ _____

Copyright 2009 First Place 4 Health. Do not duplicate without permission from First Place 4 Health.

Live It Tracker

Name: _____ Loss/gain: _____ lbs.

Date: _____ Week #: _____ Calorie Range: _____ My food goal for next week: _____

Activity Level: None, < 30 min/day, 30-60 min/day, 60+ min/day My activity goal for next week: _____

Group	Daily Calories							
	1300-1400	1500-1600	1700-1800	1900-2000	2100-2200	2300-2400	2500-2600	2700-2800
Fruits	1.5-2 c.	1.5-2 c.	1.5-2 c.	2-2.5 c.	2-2.5 c.	2.5-3.5 c.	3.5-4.5 c.	3.5-4.5 c.
Vegetables	1.5-2 c.	2-2.5 c.	2.5-3 c.	2.5-3 c.	3-3.5 c.	3.5-4.5 c.	4.5-5 c.	4.5-5 c.
Grains	5 oz-eq.	5-6 oz-eq.	6-7 oz-eq.	6-7 oz-eq.	7-8 oz-eq.	8-9 oz-eq.	9-10 oz-eq.	10-11 oz-eq.
Meat & Beans	4 oz-eq.	5 oz-eq.	5-5.5 oz-eq.	5.5-6.5 oz-eq.	6.5-7 oz-eq.	7-7.5 oz-eq.	7-7.5 oz-eq.	7.5-8 oz-eq.
Milk	2-3 c.	3 c.	3 c.	3 c.	3 c.	3 c.	3 c.	3 c.
Healthy Oils	4 tsp.	5 tsp.	5 tsp.	6 tsp.	6 tsp.	7 tsp.	8 tsp.	8 tsp.

Day/Date:

Breakfast: _____   Lunch: _____

Dinner: _____   Snack: _____

Group	Fruits	Vegetables	Grains	Meat & Beans	Milk	Oils
Goal Amount						
Estimate Your Total						
Increase ⇧ or Decrease? ⇩						

Physical Activity: _____   Spiritual Activity: _____

Steps/Miles/Minutes: _____

Day/Date:

Breakfast: _____   Lunch: _____

Dinner: _____   Snack: _____

Group	Fruits	Vegetables	Grains	Meat & Beans	Milk	Oils
Goal Amount						
Estimate Your Total						
Increase ⇧ or Decrease? ⇩						

Physical Activity: _____   Spiritual Activity: _____

Steps/Miles/Minutes: _____

Day/Date:

Breakfast: _____   Lunch: _____

Dinner: _____   Snack: _____

Group	Fruits	Vegetables	Grains	Meat & Beans	Milk	Oils
Goal Amount						
Estimate Your Total						
Increase ⇧ or Decrease? ⇩						

Physical Activity: _____   Spiritual Activity: _____

Steps/Miles/Minutes: _____

Copyright 2009 First Place 4 Health. Do not duplicate without permission from First Place 4 Health.

Day/Date:

Breakfast: _____ Lunch: _____

Dinner: _____ Snack: _____

Group	Fruits	Vegetables	Grains	Meat & Beans	Milk	Oils
Goal Amount						
Estimate Your Total						
Increase ⇧ or Decrease? ⇩						

Physical Activity: _____ Spiritual Activity: _____

Steps/Miles/Minutes: _____

Day/Date:

Breakfast: _____ Lunch: _____

Dinner: _____ Snack: _____

Group	Fruits	Vegetables	Grains	Meat & Beans	Milk	Oils
Goal Amount						
Estimate Your Total						
Increase ⇧ or Decrease? ⇩						

Physical Activity: _____ Spiritual Activity: _____

Steps/Miles/Minutes: _____

Day/Date:

Breakfast: _____ Lunch: _____

Dinner: _____ Snack: _____

Group	Fruits	Vegetables	Grains	Meat & Beans	Milk	Oils
Goal Amount						
Estimate Your Total						
Increase ⇧ or Decrease? ⇩						

Physical Activity: _____ Spiritual Activity: _____

Steps/Miles/Minutes: _____

Day/Date:

Breakfast: _____ Lunch: _____

Dinner: _____ Snack: _____

Group	Fruits	Vegetables	Grains	Meat & Beans	Milk	Oils
Goal Amount						
Estimate Your Total						
Increase ⇧ or Decrease? ⇩						

Physical Activity: _____ Spiritual Activity: _____

Steps/Miles/Minutes: _____

Copyright 2009 First Place 4 Health. Do not duplicate without permission from First Place 4 Health.

Live It Tracker

Name: _____ Loss/gain: _____ lbs.

Date: _____ Week #: _____ Calorie Range: _____ My food goal for next week: _____

Activity Level: None, < 30 min/day, 30-60 min/day, 60+ min/day My activity goal for next week: _____

Group	Daily Calories							
	1300-1400	1500-1600	1700-1800	1900-2000	2100-2200	2300-2400	2500-2600	2700-2800
Fruits	1.5-2 c.	1.5-2 c.	1.5-2 c.	2-2.5 c.	2-2.5 c.	2.5-3.5 c.	3.5-4.5 c.	3.5-4.5 c.
Vegetables	1.5-2 c.	2-2.5 c.	2.5-3 c.	2.5-3 c.	3-3.5 c.	3.5-4.5 c.	4.5-5 c.	4.5-5 c.
Grains	5 oz-eq.	5-6 oz-eq.	6-7 oz-eq.	6-7 oz-eq.	7-8 oz-eq.	8-9 oz-eq.	9-10 oz-eq.	10-11 oz-eq.
Meat & Beans	4 oz-eq.	5 oz-eq.	5-5.5 oz-eq.	5.5-6.5 oz-eq.	6.5-7 oz-eq.	7-7.5 oz-eq.	7-7.5 oz-eq.	7.5-8 oz-eq.
Milk	2-3 c.	3 c.	3 c.	3 c.	3 c.	3 c.	3 c.	3 c.
Healthy Oils	4 tsp.	5 tsp.	5 tsp.	6 tsp.	6 tsp.	7 tsp.	8 tsp.	8 tsp.

Day/Date:

Breakfast: _____ Lunch: _____

Dinner: _____ Snack: _____

Group	Fruits	Vegetables	Grains	Meat & Beans	Milk	Oils
Goal Amount						
Estimate Your Total						
Increase ⇧ or Decrease? ⇩						

Physical Activity: _____ Spiritual Activity: _____

Steps/Miles/Minutes: _____

Day/Date:

Breakfast: _____ Lunch: _____

Dinner: _____ Snack: _____

Group	Fruits	Vegetables	Grains	Meat & Beans	Milk	Oils
Goal Amount						
Estimate Your Total						
Increase ⇧ or Decrease? ⇩						

Physical Activity: _____ Spiritual Activity: _____

Steps/Miles/Minutes: _____

Day/Date:

Breakfast: _____ Lunch: _____

Dinner: _____ Snack: _____

Group	Fruits	Vegetables	Grains	Meat & Beans	Milk	Oils
Goal Amount						
Estimate Your Total						
Increase ⇧ or Decrease? ⇩						

Physical Activity: _____ Spiritual Activity: _____

Steps/Miles/Minutes: _____

Copyright 2009 First Place 4 Health. Do not duplicate without permission from First Place 4 Health.

Day/Date:

Breakfast: _____ Lunch: _____

Dinner: _____ Snack: _____

Group	Fruits	Vegetables	Grains	Meat & Beans	Milk	Oils
Goal Amount						
Estimate Your Total						
Increase ⇧ or Decrease? ⇩						

Physical Activity: _____ Spiritual Activity: _____

Steps/Miles/Minutes: _____ _____

Day/Date:

Breakfast: _____ Lunch: _____

Dinner: _____ Snack: _____

Group	Fruits	Vegetables	Grains	Meat & Beans	Milk	Oils
Goal Amount						
Estimate Your Total						
Increase ⇧ or Decrease? ⇩						

Physical Activity: _____ Spiritual Activity: _____

Steps/Miles/Minutes: _____ _____

Day/Date:

Breakfast: _____ Lunch: _____

Dinner: _____ Snack: _____

Group	Fruits	Vegetables	Grains	Meat & Beans	Milk	Oils
Goal Amount						
Estimate Your Total						
Increase ⇧ or Decrease? ⇩						

Physical Activity: _____ Spiritual Activity: _____

Steps/Miles/Minutes: _____ _____

Day/Date:

Breakfast: _____ Lunch: _____

Dinner: _____ Snack: _____

Group	Fruits	Vegetables	Grains	Meat & Beans	Milk	Oils
Goal Amount						
Estimate Your Total						
Increase ⇧ or Decrease? ⇩						

Physical Activity: _____ Spiritual Activity: _____

Steps/Miles/Minutes: _____ _____

Copyright 2009 First Place 4 Health. Do not duplicate without permission from First Place 4 Health.

Live It Tracker

Name: _____ Loss/gain: _____ lbs.

Date: _____ Week #: ____ Calorie Range: _____ My food goal for next week: _____

Activity Level: None, < 30 min/day, 30-60 min/day, 60+ min/day   My activity goal for next week: _____

Group	Daily Calories							
	1300-1400	1500-1600	1700-1800	1900-2000	2100-2200	2300-2400	2500-2600	2700-2800
Fruits	1.5-2 c.	1.5-2 c.	1.5-2 c.	2-2.5 c.	2-2.5 c.	2.5-3.5 c.	3.5-4.5 c.	3.5-4.5 c.
Vegetables	1.5-2 c.	2-2.5 c.	2.5-3 c.	2.5-3 c.	3-3.5 c.	3.5-4.5 c.	4.5-5 c.	4.5-5 c.
Grains	5 oz-eq.	5-6 oz-eq.	6-7 oz-eq.	6-7 oz-eq.	7-8 oz-eq.	8-9 oz-eq.	9-10 oz-eq.	10-11 oz-eq.
Meat & Beans	4 oz-eq.	5 oz-eq.	5-5.5 oz-eq.	5.5-6.5 oz-eq.	6.5-7 oz-eq.	7-7.5 oz-eq.	7-7.5 oz-eq.	7.5-8 oz-eq.
Milk	2-3 c.	3 c.	3 c.	3 c.	3 c.	3 c.	3 c.	3 c.
Healthy Oils	4 tsp.	5 tsp.	5 tsp.	6 tsp.	6 tsp.	7 tsp.	8 tsp.	8 tsp.

Day/Date:

Breakfast: _____   Lunch: _____

Dinner: _____   Snack: _____

Group	Fruits	Vegetables	Grains	Meat & Beans	Milk	Oils
Goal Amount						
Estimate Your Total						
Increase ⇧ or Decrease? ⇩						

Physical Activity: _____   Spiritual Activity: _____

Steps/Miles/Minutes: _____

Day/Date:

Breakfast: _____   Lunch: _____

Dinner: _____   Snack: _____

Group	Fruits	Vegetables	Grains	Meat & Beans	Milk	Oils
Goal Amount						
Estimate Your Total						
Increase ⇧ or Decrease? ⇩						

Physical Activity: _____   Spiritual Activity: _____

Steps/Miles/Minutes: _____

Day/Date:

Breakfast: _____   Lunch: _____

Dinner: _____   Snack: _____

Group	Fruits	Vegetables	Grains	Meat & Beans	Milk	Oils
Goal Amount						
Estimate Your Total						
Increase ⇧ or Decrease? ⇩						

Physical Activity: _____   Spiritual Activity: _____

Steps/Miles/Minutes: _____

Copyright 2009 First Place 4 Health. Do not duplicate without permission from First Place 4 Health.

Day/Date:

Breakfast: _____ Lunch: _____

Dinner: _____ Snack: _____

Group	Fruits	Vegetables	Grains	Meat & Beans	Milk	Oils
Goal Amount						
Estimate Your Total						
Increase ⇧ or Decrease? ⇩						

Physical Activity: _____ Spiritual Activity: _____

Steps/Miles/Minutes: _____

Day/Date:

Breakfast: _____ Lunch: _____

Dinner: _____ Snack: _____

Group	Fruits	Vegetables	Grains	Meat & Beans	Milk	Oils
Goal Amount						
Estimate Your Total						
Increase ⇧ or Decrease? ⇩						

Physical Activity: _____ Spiritual Activity: _____

Steps/Miles/Minutes: _____

Day/Date:

Breakfast: _____ Lunch: _____

Dinner: _____ Snack: _____

Group	Fruits	Vegetables	Grains	Meat & Beans	Milk	Oils
Goal Amount						
Estimate Your Total						
Increase ⇧ or Decrease? ⇩						

Physical Activity: _____ Spiritual Activity: _____

Steps/Miles/Minutes: _____

Day/Date:

Breakfast: _____ Lunch: _____

Dinner: _____ Snack: _____

Group	Fruits	Vegetables	Grains	Meat & Beans	Milk	Oils
Goal Amount						
Estimate Your Total						
Increase ⇧ or Decrease? ⇩						

Physical Activity: _____ Spiritual Activity: _____

Steps/Miles/Minutes: _____

Copyright 2009 First Place 4 Health. Do not duplicate without permission from First Place 4 Health.

Live It Tracker

Name: _____ Loss/gain: _____ lbs.

Date: _____ Week #: _____ Calorie Range: _____ My food goal for next week: _____

Activity Level: None, < 30 min/day, 30-60 min/day, 60+ min/day My activity goal for next week: _____

Group	Daily Calories							
	1300-1400	1500-1600	1700-1800	1900-2000	2100-2200	2300-2400	2500-2600	2700-2800
Fruits	1.5-2 c.	1.5-2 c.	1.5-2 c.	2-2.5 c.	2-2.5 c.	2.5-3.5 c.	3.5-4.5 c.	3.5-4.5 c.
Vegetables	1.5-2 c.	2-2.5 c.	2.5-3 c.	2.5-3 c.	3-3.5 c.	3.5-4.5 c.	4.5-5 c.	4.5-5 c.
Grains	5 oz-eq.	5-6 oz-eq.	6-7 oz-eq.	6-7 oz-eq.	7-8 oz-eq.	8-9 oz-eq.	9-10 oz-eq.	10-11 oz-eq.
Meat & Beans	4 oz-eq.	5 oz-eq.	5-5.5 oz-eq.	5.5-6.5 oz-eq.	6.5-7 oz-eq.	7-7.5 oz-eq.	7-7.5 oz-eq.	7.5-8 oz-eq.
Milk	2-3 c.	3 c.	3 c.	3 c.	3 c.	3 c.	3 c.	3 c.
Healthy Oils	4 tsp.	5 tsp.	5 tsp.	6 tsp.	6 tsp.	7 tsp.	8 tsp.	8 tsp.

Day/Date:

Breakfast: _____ Lunch: _____

Dinner: _____ Snack: _____

Group	Fruits	Vegetables	Grains	Meat & Beans	Milk	Oils
Goal Amount						
Estimate Your Total						
Increase ⇧ or Decrease? ⇩						

Physical Activity: _____ Spiritual Activity: _____

Steps/Miles/Minutes: _____

Day/Date:

Breakfast: _____ Lunch: _____

Dinner: _____ Snack: _____

Group	Fruits	Vegetables	Grains	Meat & Beans	Milk	Oils
Goal Amount						
Estimate Your Total						
Increase ⇧ or Decrease? ⇩						

Physical Activity: _____ Spiritual Activity: _____

Steps/Miles/Minutes: _____

Day/Date:

Breakfast: _____ Lunch: _____

Dinner: _____ Snack: _____

Group	Fruits	Vegetables	Grains	Meat & Beans	Milk	Oils
Goal Amount						
Estimate Your Total						
Increase ⇧ or Decrease? ⇩						

Physical Activity: _____ Spiritual Activity: _____

Steps/Miles/Minutes: _____

Copyright 2009 First Place 4 Health. Do not duplicate without permission from First Place 4 Health.

Day/Date:

Breakfast: _____   Lunch: _____

Dinner: _____   Snack: _____

Group	Fruits	Vegetables	Grains	Meat & Beans	Milk	Oils
Goal Amount						
Estimate Your Total						
Increase ⬆ or Decrease? ⬇						

Physical Activity: _____   Spiritual Activity: _____

Steps/Miles/Minutes: _____   _____

Day/Date:

Breakfast: _____   Lunch: _____

Dinner: _____   Snack: _____

Group	Fruits	Vegetables	Grains	Meat & Beans	Milk	Oils
Goal Amount						
Estimate Your Total						
Increase ⬆ or Decrease? ⬇						

Physical Activity: _____   Spiritual Activity: _____

Steps/Miles/Minutes: _____   _____

Day/Date:

Breakfast: _____   Lunch: _____

Dinner: _____   Snack: _____

Group	Fruits	Vegetables	Grains	Meat & Beans	Milk	Oils
Goal Amount						
Estimate Your Total						
Increase ⬆ or Decrease? ⬇						

Physical Activity: _____   Spiritual Activity: _____

Steps/Miles/Minutes: _____   _____

Day/Date:

Breakfast: _____   Lunch: _____

Dinner: _____   Snack: _____

Group	Fruits	Vegetables	Grains	Meat & Beans	Milk	Oils
Goal Amount						
Estimate Your Total						
Increase ⬆ or Decrease? ⬇						

Physical Activity: _____   Spiritual Activity: _____

Steps/Miles/Minutes: _____   _____

Copyright 2009 First Place 4 Health. Do not duplicate without permission from First Place 4 Health.

Live It Tracker

Name: _____ Loss/gain: _____ lbs.

Date: _____ Week #: _____ Calorie Range: _____ My food goal for next week: _____

Activity Level: None, < 30 min/day, 30-60 min/day, 60+ min/day My activity goal for next week: _____

Group	Daily Calories							
	1300-1400	1500-1600	1700-1800	1900-2000	2100-2200	2300-2400	2500-2600	2700-2800
Fruits	1.5-2 c.	1.5-2 c.	1.5-2 c.	2-2.5 c.	2-2.5 c.	2.5-3.5 c.	3.5-4.5 c.	3.5-4.5 c.
Vegetables	1.5-2 c.	2-2.5 c.	2.5-3 c.	2.5-3 c.	3-3.5 c.	3.5-4.5 c.	4.5-5 c.	4.5-5 c.
Grains	5 oz-eq.	5-6 oz-eq.	6-7 oz-eq.	6-7 oz-eq.	7-8 oz-eq.	8-9 oz-eq.	9-10 oz-eq.	10-11 oz-eq.
Meat & Beans	4 oz-eq.	5 oz-eq.	5-5.5 oz-eq.	5.5-6.5 oz-eq.	6.5-7 oz-eq.	7-7.5 oz-eq.	7-7.5 oz-eq.	7.5-8 oz-eq.
Milk	2-3 c.	3 c.	3 c.	3 c.	3 c.	3 c.	3 c.	3 c.
Healthy Oils	4 tsp.	5 tsp.	5 tsp.	6 tsp.	6 tsp.	7 tsp.	8 tsp.	8 tsp.

Day/Date: _____

Breakfast: _____ Lunch: _____

Dinner: _____ Snack: _____

Group	Fruits	Vegetables	Grains	Meat & Beans	Milk	Oils
Goal Amount						
Estimate Your Total						
Increase ⇧ or Decrease? ⇩						

Physical Activity: _____ Spiritual Activity: _____

Steps/Miles/Minutes: _____

Day/Date: _____

Breakfast: _____ Lunch: _____

Dinner: _____ Snack: _____

Group	Fruits	Vegetables	Grains	Meat & Beans	Milk	Oils
Goal Amount						
Estimate Your Total						
Increase ⇧ or Decrease? ⇩						

Physical Activity: _____ Spiritual Activity: _____

Steps/Miles/Minutes: _____

Day/Date: _____

Breakfast: _____ Lunch: _____

Dinner: _____ Snack: _____

Group	Fruits	Vegetables	Grains	Meat & Beans	Milk	Oils
Goal Amount						
Estimate Your Total						
Increase ⇧ or Decrease? ⇩						

Physical Activity: _____ Spiritual Activity: _____

Steps/Miles/Minutes: _____

Copyright 2009 First Place 4 Health. Do not duplicate without permission from First Place 4 Health.

Day/Date:

Breakfast: _____ Lunch: _____

Dinner: _____ Snack: _____

Group	Fruits	Vegetables	Grains	Meat & Beans	Milk	Oils
Goal Amount						
Estimate Your Total						
Increase ⇧ or Decrease? ⇩						

Physical Activity: _____ Spiritual Activity: _____

Steps/Miles/Minutes: _____ _____

Day/Date:

Breakfast: _____ Lunch: _____

Dinner: _____ Snack: _____

Group	Fruits	Vegetables	Grains	Meat & Beans	Milk	Oils
Goal Amount						
Estimate Your Total						
Increase ⇧ or Decrease? ⇩						

Physical Activity: _____ Spiritual Activity: _____

Steps/Miles/Minutes: _____ _____

Day/Date:

Breakfast: _____ Lunch: _____

Dinner: _____ Snack: _____

Group	Fruits	Vegetables	Grains	Meat & Beans	Milk	Oils
Goal Amount						
Estimate Your Total						
Increase ⇧ or Decrease? ⇩						

Physical Activity: _____ Spiritual Activity: _____

Steps/Miles/Minutes: _____ _____

Day/Date:

Breakfast: _____ Lunch: _____

Dinner: _____ Snack: _____

Group	Fruits	Vegetables	Grains	Meat & Beans	Milk	Oils
Goal Amount						
Estimate Your Total						
Increase ⇧ or Decrease? ⇩						

Physical Activity: _____ Spiritual Activity: _____

Steps/Miles/Minutes: _____ _____

Copyright 2009 First Place 4 Health. Do not duplicate without permission from First Place 4 Health.

Live It Tracker

Name: _____ Loss/gain: _____ lbs.

Date: _____ Week #: _____ Calorie Range: _____ My food goal for next week: _____

Activity Level: None, < 30 min/day, 30-60 min/day, 60+ min/day My activity goal for next week: _____

Group	Daily Calories							
	1300-1400	1500-1600	1700-1800	1900-2000	2100-2200	2300-2400	2500-2600	2700-2800
Fruits	1.5-2 c.	1.5-2 c.	1.5-2 c.	2-2.5 c.	2-2.5 c.	2.5-3.5 c.	3.5-4.5 c.	3.5-4.5 c.
Vegetables	1.5-2 c.	2-2.5 c.	2.5-3 c.	2.5-3 c.	3-3.5 c.	3.5-4.5 c.	4.5-5 c.	4.5-5 c.
Grains	5 oz-eq.	5-6 oz-eq.	6-7 oz-eq.	6-7 oz-eq.	7-8 oz-eq.	8-9 oz-eq.	9-10 oz-eq.	10-11 oz-eq.
Meat & Beans	4 oz-eq.	5 oz-eq.	5-5.5 oz-eq.	5.5-6.5 oz-eq.	6.5-7 oz-eq.	7-7.5 oz-eq.	7-7.5 oz-eq.	7.5-8 oz-eq.
Milk	2-3 c.	3 c.	3 c.	3 c.	3 c.	3 c.	3 c.	3 c.
Healthy Oils	4 tsp.	5 tsp.	5 tsp.	6 tsp.	6 tsp.	7 tsp.	8 tsp.	8 tsp.

Day/Date:

Breakfast: _____ Lunch: _____

Dinner: _____ Snack: _____

Group	Fruits	Vegetables	Grains	Meat & Beans	Milk	Oils
Goal Amount						
Estimate Your Total						
Increase ⬆ or Decrease? ⬇						

Physical Activity: _____ Spiritual Activity: _____

Steps/Miles/Minutes: _____

Day/Date:

Breakfast: _____ Lunch: _____

Dinner: _____ Snack: _____

Group	Fruits	Vegetables	Grains	Meat & Beans	Milk	Oils
Goal Amount						
Estimate Your Total						
Increase ⬆ or Decrease? ⬇						

Physical Activity: _____ Spiritual Activity: _____

Steps/Miles/Minutes: _____

Day/Date:

Breakfast: _____ Lunch: _____

Dinner: _____ Snack: _____

Group	Fruits	Vegetables	Grains	Meat & Beans	Milk	Oils
Goal Amount						
Estimate Your Total						
Increase ⬆ or Decrease? ⬇						

Physical Activity: _____ Spiritual Activity: _____

Steps/Miles/Minutes: _____

Copyright 2009 First Place 4 Health. Do not duplicate without permission from First Place 4 Health.

Day/Date:

Breakfast: _____ Lunch: _____

Dinner: _____ Snack: _____

Group	Fruits	Vegetables	Grains	Meat & Beans	Milk	Oils
Goal Amount						
Estimate Your Total						
Increase ⇧ or Decrease? ⇩						

Physical Activity: _____ Spiritual Activity: _____

Steps/Miles/Minutes: _____ _____

Day/Date:

Breakfast: _____ Lunch: _____

Dinner: _____ Snack: _____

Group	Fruits	Vegetables	Grains	Meat & Beans	Milk	Oils
Goal Amount						
Estimate Your Total						
Increase ⇧ or Decrease? ⇩						

Physical Activity: _____ Spiritual Activity: _____

Steps/Miles/Minutes: _____ _____

Day/Date:

Breakfast: _____ Lunch: _____

Dinner: _____ Snack: _____

Group	Fruits	Vegetables	Grains	Meat & Beans	Milk	Oils
Goal Amount						
Estimate Your Total						
Increase ⇧ or Decrease? ⇩						

Physical Activity: _____ Spiritual Activity: _____

Steps/Miles/Minutes: _____ _____

Day/Date:

Breakfast: _____ Lunch: _____

Dinner: _____ Snack: _____

Group	Fruits	Vegetables	Grains	Meat & Beans	Milk	Oils
Goal Amount						
Estimate Your Total						
Increase ⇧ or Decrease? ⇩						

Physical Activity: _____ Spiritual Activity: _____

Steps/Miles/Minutes: _____ _____

Copyright 2009 First Place 4 Health. Do not duplicate without permission from First Place 4 Health.

Live It Tracker

Name: _____ Loss/gain: _____ lbs.

Date: _____ Week #: _____ Calorie Range: _____ My food goal for next week: _____

Activity Level: None, < 30 min/day, 30-60 min/day, 60+ min/day My activity goal for next week: _____

Group	Daily Calories							
	1300-1400	1500-1600	1700-1800	1900-2000	2100-2200	2300-2400	2500-2600	2700-2800
Fruits	1.5-2 c.	1.5-2 c.	1.5-2 c.	2-2.5 c.	2-2.5 c.	2.5-3.5 c.	3.5-4.5 c.	3.5-4.5 c.
Vegetables	1.5-2 c.	2-2.5 c.	2.5-3 c.	2.5-3 c.	3-3.5 c.	3.5-4.5 c.	4.5-5 c.	4.5-5 c.
Grains	5 oz-eq.	5-6 oz-eq.	6-7 oz-eq.	6-7 oz-eq.	7-8 oz-eq.	8-9 oz-eq.	9-10 oz-eq.	10-11 oz-eq.
Meat & Beans	4 oz-eq.	5 oz-eq.	5-5.5 oz-eq.	5.5-6.5 oz-eq.	6.5-7 oz-eq.	7-7.5 oz-eq.	7-7.5 oz-eq.	7.5-8 oz-eq.
Milk	2-3 c.	3 c.	3 c.	3 c.	3 c.	3 c.	3 c.	3 c.
Healthy Oils	4 tsp.	5 tsp.	5 tsp.	6 tsp.	6 tsp.	7 tsp.	8 tsp.	8 tsp.

Day/Date:

Breakfast: _____ Lunch: _____

Dinner: _____ Snack: _____

Group	Fruits	Vegetables	Grains	Meat & Beans	Milk	Oils
Goal Amount						
Estimate Your Total						
Increase ⇧ or Decrease? ⇩						

Physical Activity: _____ Spiritual Activity: _____

Steps/Miles/Minutes: _____

Day/Date:

Breakfast: _____ Lunch: _____

Dinner: _____ Snack: _____

Group	Fruits	Vegetables	Grains	Meat & Beans	Milk	Oils
Goal Amount						
Estimate Your Total						
Increase ⇧ or Decrease? ⇩						

Physical Activity: _____ Spiritual Activity: _____

Steps/Miles/Minutes: _____

Day/Date:

Breakfast: _____ Lunch: _____

Dinner: _____ Snack: _____

Group	Fruits	Vegetables	Grains	Meat & Beans	Milk	Oils
Goal Amount						
Estimate Your Total						
Increase ⇧ or Decrease? ⇩						

Physical Activity: _____ Spiritual Activity: _____

Steps/Miles/Minutes: _____

Copyright 2009 First Place 4 Health. Do not duplicate without permission from First Place 4 Health.

Day/Date: _____

Breakfast: _____ Lunch: _____

Dinner: _____ Snack: _____

Group	Fruits	Vegetables	Grains	Meat & Beans	Milk	Oils
Goal Amount						
Estimate Your Total						
Increase ⇧ or Decrease? ⇩						

Physical Activity: _____ Spiritual Activity: _____

Steps/Miles/Minutes: _____ _____

Day/Date: _____

Breakfast: _____ Lunch: _____

Dinner: _____ Snack: _____

Group	Fruits	Vegetables	Grains	Meat & Beans	Milk	Oils
Goal Amount						
Estimate Your Total						
Increase ⇧ or Decrease? ⇩						

Physical Activity: _____ Spiritual Activity: _____

Steps/Miles/Minutes: _____ _____

Day/Date: _____

Breakfast: _____ Lunch: _____

Dinner: _____ Snack: _____

Group	Fruits	Vegetables	Grains	Meat & Beans	Milk	Oils
Goal Amount						
Estimate Your Total						
Increase ⇧ or Decrease? ⇩						

Physical Activity: _____ Spiritual Activity: _____

Steps/Miles/Minutes: _____ _____

Day/Date: _____

Breakfast: _____ Lunch: _____

Dinner: _____ Snack: _____

Group	Fruits	Vegetables	Grains	Meat & Beans	Milk	Oils
Goal Amount						
Estimate Your Total						
Increase ⇧ or Decrease? ⇩						

Physical Activity: _____ Spiritual Activity: _____

Steps/Miles/Minutes: _____ _____

Copyright 2009 First Place 4 Health. Do not duplicate without permission from First Place 4 Health.

Live It Tracker

Name: _____ Loss/gain: _____ lbs.

Date: _____ Week #: _____ Calorie Range: _____ My food goal for next week: _____

Activity Level: None, < 30 min/day, 30-60 min/day, 60+ min/day My activity goal for next week: _____

Group	Daily Calories							
	1300-1400	1500-1600	1700-1800	1900-2000	2100-2200	2300-2400	2500-2600	2700-2800
Fruits	1.5-2 c.	1.5-2 c.	1.5-2 c.	2-2.5 c.	2-2.5 c.	2.5-3.5 c.	3.5-4.5 c.	3.5-4.5 c.
Vegetables	1.5-2 c.	2-2.5 c.	2.5-3 c.	2.5-3 c.	3-3.5 c.	3.5-4.5 c.	4.5-5 c.	4.5-5 c.
Grains	5 oz-eq.	5-6 oz-eq.	6-7 oz-eq.	6-7 oz-eq.	7-8 oz-eq.	8-9 oz-eq.	9-10 oz-eq.	10-11 oz-eq.
Meat & Beans	4 oz-eq.	5 oz-eq.	5-5.5 oz-eq.	5.5-6.5 oz-eq.	6.5-7 oz-eq.	7-7.5 oz-eq.	7-7.5 oz-eq.	7.5-8 oz-eq.
Milk	2-3 c.	3 c.	3 c.	3 c.	3 c.	3 c.	3 c.	3 c.
Healthy Oils	4 tsp.	5 tsp.	5 tsp.	6 tsp.	6 tsp.	7 tsp.	8 tsp.	8 tsp.

Day/Date:

Breakfast: _____ Lunch: _____

Dinner: _____ Snack: _____

Group	Fruits	Vegetables	Grains	Meat & Beans	Milk	Oils
Goal Amount						
Estimate Your Total						
Increase ⇧ or Decrease? ⇩						

Physical Activity: _____ Spiritual Activity: _____

Steps/Miles/Minutes: _____

Day/Date:

Breakfast: _____ Lunch: _____

Dinner: _____ Snack: _____

Group	Fruits	Vegetables	Grains	Meat & Beans	Milk	Oils
Goal Amount						
Estimate Your Total						
Increase ⇧ or Decrease? ⇩						

Physical Activity: _____ Spiritual Activity: _____

Steps/Miles/Minutes: _____

Day/Date:

Breakfast: _____ Lunch: _____

Dinner: _____ Snack: _____

Group	Fruits	Vegetables	Grains	Meat & Beans	Milk	Oils
Goal Amount						
Estimate Your Total						
Increase ⇧ or Decrease? ⇩						

Physical Activity: _____ Spiritual Activity: _____

Steps/Miles/Minutes: _____

Copyright 2009 First Place 4 Health. Do not duplicate without permission from First Place 4 Health.

Day/Date: ___

Breakfast: _____ Lunch: _____

Dinner: _____ Snack: _____

Group	Fruits	Vegetables	Grains	Meat & Beans	Milk	Oils
Goal Amount						
Estimate Your Total						
Increase ⇧ or Decrease? ⇩						

Physical Activity: _____ Spiritual Activity: _____

Steps/Miles/Minutes: _____ _____

Day/Date: ___

Breakfast: _____ Lunch: _____

Dinner: _____ Snack: _____

Group	Fruits	Vegetables	Grains	Meat & Beans	Milk	Oils
Goal Amount						
Estimate Your Total						
Increase ⇧ or Decrease? ⇩						

Physical Activity: _____ Spiritual Activity: _____

Steps/Miles/Minutes: _____ _____

Day/Date: ___

Breakfast: _____ Lunch: _____

Dinner: _____ Snack: _____

Group	Fruits	Vegetables	Grains	Meat & Beans	Milk	Oils
Goal Amount						
Estimate Your Total						
Increase ⇧ or Decrease? ⇩						

Physical Activity: _____ Spiritual Activity: _____

Steps/Miles/Minutes: _____ _____

Day/Date: ___

Breakfast: _____ Lunch: _____

Dinner: _____ Snack: _____

Group	Fruits	Vegetables	Grains	Meat & Beans	Milk	Oils
Goal Amount						
Estimate Your Total						
Increase ⇧ or Decrease? ⇩						

Physical Activity: _____ Spiritual Activity: _____

Steps/Miles/Minutes: _____ _____

Copyright 2009 First Place 4 Health. Do not duplicate without permission from First Place 4 Health.

Live It Tracker

Name: _____ Loss/gain: _____ lbs.

Date: _____ Week #: _____ Calorie Range: _____ My food goal for next week: _____

Activity Level: None, < 30 min/day, 30-60 min/day, 60+ min/day My activity goal for next week: _____

Group	Daily Calories							
	1300-1400	1500-1600	1700-1800	1900-2000	2100-2200	2300-2400	2500-2600	2700-2800
Fruits	1.5-2 c.	1.5-2 c.	1.5-2 c.	2-2.5 c.	2-2.5 c.	2.5-3.5 c.	3.5-4.5 c.	3.5-4.5 c.
Vegetables	1.5-2 c.	2-2.5 c.	2.5-3 c.	2.5-3 c.	3-3.5 c.	3.5-4.5 c.	4.5-5 c.	4.5-5 c.
Grains	5 oz-eq.	5-6 oz-eq.	6-7 oz-eq.	6-7 oz-eq.	7-8 oz-eq.	8-9 oz-eq.	9-10 oz-eq.	10-11 oz-eq.
Meat & Beans	4 oz-eq.	5 oz-eq.	5-5.5 oz-eq.	5.5-6.5 oz-eq.	6.5-7 oz-eq.	7-7.5 oz-eq.	7-7.5 oz-eq.	7.5-8 oz-eq.
Milk	2-3 c.	3 c.	3 c.	3 c.	3 c.	3 c.	3 c.	3 c.
Healthy Oils	4 tsp.	5 tsp.	5 tsp.	6 tsp.	6 tsp.	7 tsp.	8 tsp.	8 tsp.

Day/Date:

Breakfast: _____   Lunch: _____

Dinner: _____   Snack: _____

Group	Fruits	Vegetables	Grains	Meat & Beans	Milk	Oils
Goal Amount						
Estimate Your Total						
Increase ⇧ or Decrease? ⇩						

Physical Activity: _____   Spiritual Activity: _____

Steps/Miles/Minutes: _____

Day/Date:

Breakfast: _____   Lunch: _____

Dinner: _____   Snack: _____

Group	Fruits	Vegetables	Grains	Meat & Beans	Milk	Oils
Goal Amount						
Estimate Your Total						
Increase ⇧ or Decrease? ⇩						

Physical Activity: _____   Spiritual Activity: _____

Steps/Miles/Minutes: _____

Day/Date:

Breakfast: _____   Lunch: _____

Dinner: _____   Snack: _____

Group	Fruits	Vegetables	Grains	Meat & Beans	Milk	Oils
Goal Amount						
Estimate Your Total						
Increase ⇧ or Decrease? ⇩						

Physical Activity: _____   Spiritual Activity: _____

Steps/Miles/Minutes: _____

Copyright 2009 First Place 4 Health. Do not duplicate without permission from First Place 4 Health.

Day/Date:

Breakfast: _____   Lunch: _____

Dinner: _____   Snack: _____

Group	Fruits	Vegetables	Grains	Meat & Beans	Milk	Oils
Goal Amount						
Estimate Your Total						
Increase ⇧ or Decrease? ⇩						

Physical Activity: _____   Spiritual Activity: _____

Steps/Miles/Minutes: _____

Day/Date:

Breakfast: _____   Lunch: _____

Dinner: _____   Snack: _____

Group	Fruits	Vegetables	Grains	Meat & Beans	Milk	Oils
Goal Amount						
Estimate Your Total						
Increase ⇧ or Decrease? ⇩						

Physical Activity: _____   Spiritual Activity: _____

Steps/Miles/Minutes: _____

Day/Date:

Breakfast: _____   Lunch: _____

Dinner: _____   Snack: _____

Group	Fruits	Vegetables	Grains	Meat & Beans	Milk	Oils
Goal Amount						
Estimate Your Total						
Increase ⇧ or Decrease? ⇩						

Physical Activity: _____   Spiritual Activity: _____

Steps/Miles/Minutes: _____

Day/Date:

Breakfast: _____   Lunch: _____

Dinner: _____   Snack: _____

Group	Fruits	Vegetables	Grains	Meat & Beans	Milk	Oils
Goal Amount						
Estimate Your Total						
Increase ⇧ or Decrease? ⇩						

Physical Activity: _____   Spiritual Activity: _____

Steps/Miles/Minutes: _____

Copyright 2009 First Place 4 Health. Do not duplicate without permission from First Place 4 Health.

Live It Tracker

Name: _____ Loss/gain: _____ lbs.

Date: _____ Week #: _____ Calorie Range: _____ My food goal for next week: _____

Activity Level: None, < 30 min/day, 30-60 min/day, 60+ min/day My activity goal for next week: _____

Group	Daily Calories							
	1300-1400	1500-1600	1700-1800	1900-2000	2100-2200	2300-2400	2500-2600	2700-2800
Fruits	1.5-2 c.	1.5-2 c.	1.5-2 c.	2-2.5 c.	2-2.5 c.	2.5-3.5 c.	3.5-4.5 c.	3.5-4.5 c.
Vegetables	1.5-2 c.	2-2.5 c.	2.5-3 c.	2.5-3 c.	3-3.5 c.	3.5-4.5 c.	4.5-5 c.	4.5-5 c.
Grains	5 oz-eq.	5-6 oz-eq.	6-7 oz-eq.	6-7 oz-eq.	7-8 oz-eq.	8-9 oz-eq.	9-10 oz-eq.	10-11 oz-eq.
Meat & Beans	4 oz-eq.	5 oz-eq.	5-5.5 oz-eq.	5.5-6.5 oz-eq.	6.5-7 oz-eq.	7-7.5 oz-eq.	7-7.5 oz-eq.	7.5-8 oz-eq.
Milk	2-3 c.	3 c.	3 c.	3 c.	3 c.	3 c.	3 c.	3 c.
Healthy Oils	4 tsp.	5 tsp.	5 tsp.	6 tsp.	6 tsp.	7 tsp.	8 tsp.	8 tsp.

Day/Date: _____

Breakfast: _____ Lunch: _____

Dinner: _____ Snack: _____

Group	Fruits	Vegetables	Grains	Meat & Beans	Milk	Oils
Goal Amount						
Estimate Your Total						
Increase ⇧ or Decrease? ⇩						

Physical Activity: _____ Spiritual Activity: _____

Steps/Miles/Minutes: _____

Day/Date: _____

Breakfast: _____ Lunch: _____

Dinner: _____ Snack: _____

Group	Fruits	Vegetables	Grains	Meat & Beans	Milk	Oils
Goal Amount						
Estimate Your Total						
Increase ⇧ or Decrease? ⇩						

Physical Activity: _____ Spiritual Activity: _____

Steps/Miles/Minutes: _____

Day/Date: _____

Breakfast: _____ Lunch: _____

Dinner: _____ Snack: _____

Group	Fruits	Vegetables	Grains	Meat & Beans	Milk	Oils
Goal Amount						
Estimate Your Total						
Increase ⇧ or Decrease? ⇩						

Physical Activity: _____ Spiritual Activity: _____

Steps/Miles/Minutes: _____

Copyright 2009 First Place 4 Health. Do not duplicate without permission from First Place 4 Health.

Day/Date: _____

Breakfast: _____ Lunch: _____

Dinner: _____ Snack: _____

Group	Fruits	Vegetables	Grains	Meat & Beans	Milk	Oils
Goal Amount						
Estimate Your Total						
Increase ⇧ or Decrease? ⇩						

Physical Activity: _____ Spiritual Activity: _____

Steps/Miles/Minutes: _____ _____

Day/Date: _____

Breakfast: _____ Lunch: _____

Dinner: _____ Snack: _____

Group	Fruits	Vegetables	Grains	Meat & Beans	Milk	Oils
Goal Amount						
Estimate Your Total						
Increase ⇧ or Decrease? ⇩						

Physical Activity: _____ Spiritual Activity: _____

Steps/Miles/Minutes: _____ _____

Day/Date: _____

Breakfast: _____ Lunch: _____

Dinner: _____ Snack: _____

Group	Fruits	Vegetables	Grains	Meat & Beans	Milk	Oils
Goal Amount						
Estimate Your Total						
Increase ⇧ or Decrease? ⇩						

Physical Activity: _____ Spiritual Activity: _____

Steps/Miles/Minutes: _____ _____

Day/Date: _____

Breakfast: _____ Lunch: _____

Dinner: _____ Snack: _____

Group	Fruits	Vegetables	Grains	Meat & Beans	Milk	Oils
Goal Amount						
Estimate Your Total						
Increase ⇧ or Decrease? ⇩						

Physical Activity: _____ Spiritual Activity: _____

Steps/Miles/Minutes: _____ _____

Copyright 2009 First Place 4 Health. Do not duplicate without permission from First Place 4 Health.

Live It Tracker

Name: _____ Loss/gain: _____ lbs.

Date: _____ Week #: _____ Calorie Range: _____ My food goal for next week: _____

Activity Level: None, < 30 min/day, 30-60 min/day, 60+ min/day My activity goal for next week: _____

Group	Daily Calories							
	1300-1400	1500-1600	1700-1800	1900-2000	2100-2200	2300-2400	2500-2600	2700-2800
Fruits	1.5-2 c.	1.5-2 c.	1.5-2 c.	2-2.5 c.	2-2.5 c.	2.5-3.5 c.	3.5-4.5 c.	3.5-4.5 c.
Vegetables	1.5-2 c.	2-2.5 c.	2.5-3 c.	2.5-3 c.	3-3.5 c.	3.5-4.5 c.	4.5-5 c.	4.5-5 c.
Grains	5 oz-eq.	5-6 oz-eq.	6-7 oz-eq.	6-7 oz-eq.	7-8 oz-eq.	8-9 oz-eq.	9-10 oz-eq.	10-11 oz-eq.
Meat & Beans	4 oz-eq.	5 oz-eq.	5-5.5 oz-eq.	5.5-6.5 oz-eq.	6.5-7 oz-eq.	7-7.5 oz-eq.	7-7.5 oz-eq.	7.5-8 oz-eq.
Milk	2-3 c.	3 c.	3 c.	3 c.	3 c.	3 c.	3 c.	3 c.
Healthy Oils	4 tsp.	5 tsp.	5 tsp.	6 tsp.	6 tsp.	7 tsp.	8 tsp.	8 tsp.

Day/Date:

Breakfast: _____ Lunch: _____

Dinner: _____ Snack: _____

Group	Fruits	Vegetables	Grains	Meat & Beans	Milk	Oils
Goal Amount						
Estimate Your Total						
Increase ⇧ or Decrease? ⇩						

Physical Activity: _____ Spiritual Activity: _____

Steps/Miles/Minutes: _____

Day/Date:

Breakfast: _____ Lunch: _____

Dinner: _____ Snack: _____

Group	Fruits	Vegetables	Grains	Meat & Beans	Milk	Oils
Goal Amount						
Estimate Your Total						
Increase ⇧ or Decrease? ⇩						

Physical Activity: _____ Spiritual Activity: _____

Steps/Miles/Minutes: _____

Day/Date:

Breakfast: _____ Lunch: _____

Dinner: _____ Snack: _____

Group	Fruits	Vegetables	Grains	Meat & Beans	Milk	Oils
Goal Amount						
Estimate Your Total						
Increase ⇧ or Decrease? ⇩						

Physical Activity: _____ Spiritual Activity: _____

Steps/Miles/Minutes: _____

Copyright 2009 First Place 4 Health. Do not duplicate without permission from First Place 4 Health.

Breakfast: _____ **Lunch:** _____

Dinner: _____ **Snack:** _____

Group	Fruits	Vegetables	Grains	Meat & Beans	Milk	Oils
Goal Amount						
Estimate Your Total						
Increase ⇧ or Decrease? ⇩						

Physical Activity: _____ **Spiritual Activity:** _____

Steps/Miles/Minutes: _____ _____

Breakfast: _____ **Lunch:** _____

Dinner: _____ **Snack:** _____

Group	Fruits	Vegetables	Grains	Meat & Beans	Milk	Oils
Goal Amount						
Estimate Your Total						
Increase ⇧ or Decrease? ⇩						

Physical Activity: _____ **Spiritual Activity:** _____

Steps/Miles/Minutes: _____ _____

Breakfast: _____ **Lunch:** _____

Dinner: _____ **Snack:** _____

Group	Fruits	Vegetables	Grains	Meat & Beans	Milk	Oils
Goal Amount						
Estimate Your Total						
Increase ⇧ or Decrease? ⇩						

Physical Activity: _____ **Spiritual Activity:** _____

Steps/Miles/Minutes: _____ _____

Breakfast: _____ **Lunch:** _____

Dinner: _____ **Snack:** _____

Group	Fruits	Vegetables	Grains	Meat & Beans	Milk	Oils
Goal Amount						
Estimate Your Total						
Increase ⇧ or Decrease? ⇩						

Physical Activity: _____ **Spiritual Activity:** _____

Steps/Miles/Minutes: _____ _____

Copyright 2009 First Place 4 Health. Do not duplicate without permission from First Place 4 Health.

let's count our miles!

Join the 100-Mile Club this Session

Can't walk that mile yet? Don't be discouraged! There are exercises you can do to strengthen your body and burn those extra calories. Keep a record on your Live It Tracker of the number of minutes you do these common physical activities, convert those minutes to miles following the chart below, and then mark off each mile you have completed on the chart found on the back of the front cover. Report your miles to your 100-Mile Club representative when you first arrive each week. Remember, you are not competing with anyone else . . . just yourself. Your job is to strive to reach 100 miles before the last meeting in this session. You can do it—just keep on moving!

Walking
slowly, 2 mph	30 min. = 156 cal. = 1 mile
moderately, 3 mph	20 min. = 156 cal. = 1 mile
very briskly, 4 mph	15 min. = 156 cal. = 1 mile
speed walking	10 min. = 156 cal. = 1 mile
up stairs	13 min. = 159 cal. = 1 mile

Running/Jogging
10 min. = 156 cal. = 1 mile

Cycling Outdoors
slowly, <10 mph	20 min. = 156 cal. = 1 mile
light effort, 10-12 mph	12 min. = 156 cal. = 1 mile
moderate effort, 12-14 mph	10 min. = 156 cal. = 1 mile
vigorous effort, 14-16 mph	7.5 min. = 156 cal. = 1 mile
very fast, 16 19 mph	6.5 min = 152 cal. = 1 mile

Sports Activities
Playing tennis (singles)	10 min. = 156 cal. = 1 mile
Swimming	
light to moderate effort	11 min. = 152 cal. = 1 mile
fast, vigorous effort	7.5 min. = 156 cal. = 1 mile
Softball	15 min. = 156 cal. = 1 mile
Golf	20 min. = 156 cal = 1 mile
Rollerblading	6.5 min. = 152 cal. = 1 mile
Ice skating	11 min. = 152 cal. = 1 mile

Jumping rope	7.5 min. = 156 cal. = 1 mile
Basketball	12 min. = 156 cal. = 1 mile
Soccer (casual)	15 min. = 159 cal. = 1 mile

Around the House

Mowing grass	22 min. = 156 cal. = 1 mile
Mopping, sweeping, vacuuming	19.5 min. = 155 cal. = 1 mile
Cooking	40 min. =160 cal. = 1 mile
Gardening	19 min. = 156 cal. = 1 mile
Housework (general)	35 min. = 156 cal. = 1 mile
Ironing	45 min. = 153 cal. = 1 mile
Raking leaves	25 min. = 150 cal. = 1 mile
Washing car	23 min. = 156 cal. = 1 mile
Washing dishes	45 min. = 153 cal. = 1 mile

At the Gym

Stair machine	8.5 min. = 155 cal. = 1 mile
Stationary bike	
slowly, 10 mph	30 min. = 156 cal. = 1 mile
moderately, 10-13 mph	15 min. = 156 cal. = 1 mile
vigorously, 13-16 mph	7.5 min. = 156 cal. = 1 mile
briskly, 16-19 mph	6.5 min. = 156 cal. = 1 mile
Elliptical trainer	12 min. = 156 cal. = 1 mile
Weight machines (used vigorously)	13 min. = 152 cal.=1 mile
Aerobics	
low impact	15 min. = 156 cal. = 1 mile
high impact	12 min. = 156 cal. = 1 mile
water	20 min. = 156 cal. = 1 mile
Pilates	15 min. = 156 cal. = 1 mile
Raquetball (casual)	15 min. = 159 cal. = 1 mile
Stretching exercises	25 min. = 150 cal. = 1 mile
Weight lifting (also works for weight machines used moderately or gently)	30 min. = 156 cal. = 1 mile

Family Leisure

Playing piano	37 min. = 155 cal. = 1 mile
Jumping rope	10 min. = 152 cal. = 1 mile
Skating (moderate)	20 min. = 152 cal. = 1 mile
Swimming	
moderate	17 min. = 156 cal. = 1 mile
vigorous	10 min. = 148 cal. = 1 mile
Table tennis	25 min. = 150 cal. = 1 mile
Walk/run/play with kids	25 min. = 150 cal. = 1 mile